the POST-MENOPAUSE *method*

the POST-MENOPAUSE *method*

A nutritional guide to ageing well

KAREN NEWBY

PAVILION

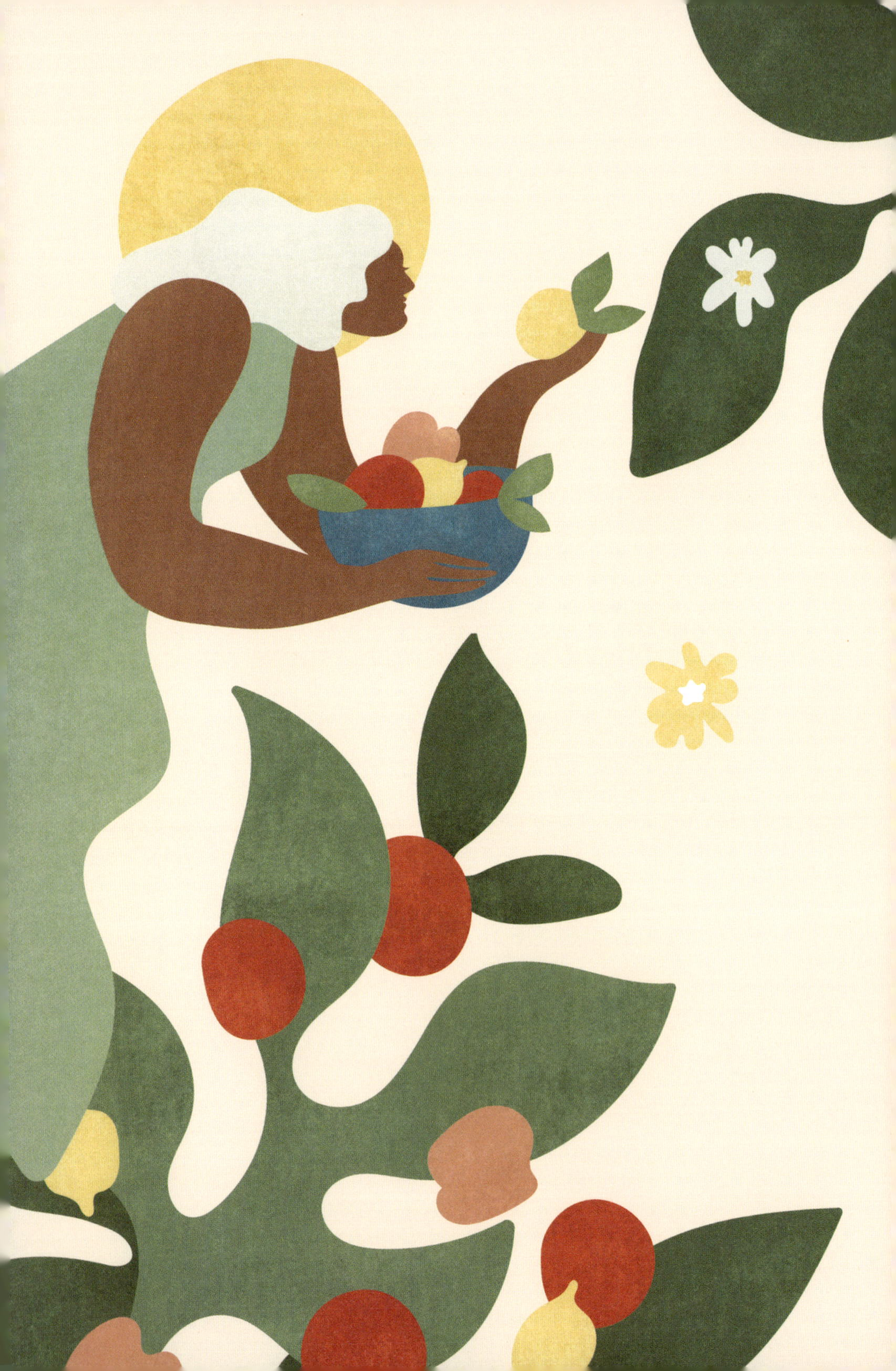

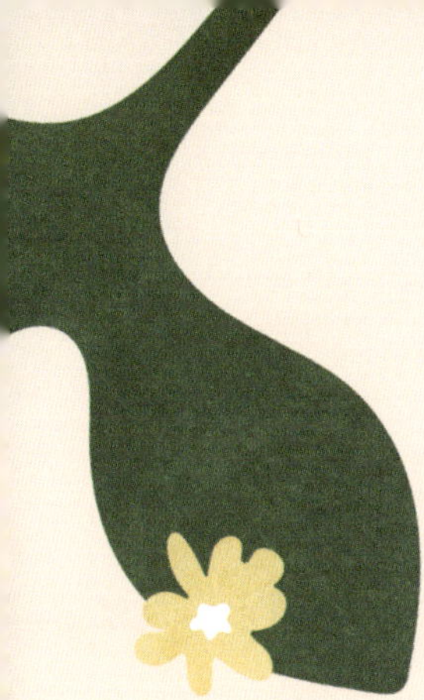

Contents

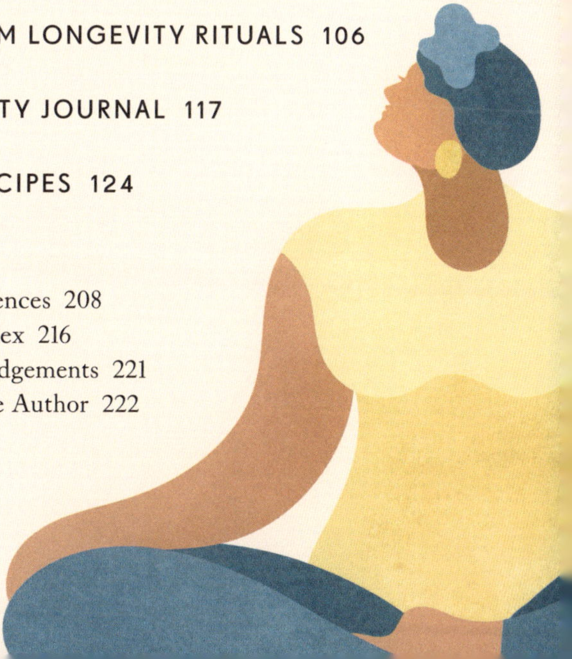

introduction

A FEMALE APPROACH TO LONGEVITY

Do you want to live forever? When I ask this question at speaking events most women will say no. We don't want to live until we're 120, like the longevity biohacking bros do (I'm not even sure they actually look that happy or healthy either!), but what we do want is to lead lives full of vitality, connection and community, and without chronic disease for as long as possible. For those struggling with illness, I hope this book will be a helpful companion, equipping you for healing or for dealing with a longer-term condition. This book is entirely dedicated to helping you all achieve a life filled with energy and purpose.

We do have agency over our health, post-menopause, but when we are bombarded with scare stories about our health dropping off a cliff (don't get me wrong – our risk factors for certain diseases do go up), it can all seem rather overwhelming. This includes stories such as, 'If you're not on HRT your brain will shrink', which is clearly a terrifying (and completely unfounded) message for those of us not on HRT, like me. We are also grappling with a booming wellness industry, and within that, the rapidly expanding longevity industry, which has got very good at creating problems that we didn't know we had, accompanied by costly solutions. Unfortunately, meno-washing and wellness-washing products take the focus away from genuine health-supporting rituals in favour of the shiny new longevity products and gadgets offering false promises of long health and vitality.

All of this 'wellness noise' is very far removed from what the most extraordinary and longest-living women on the planet do, such as those living on the island of Okinawa, Japan. These women naturally follow the longevity patterns outlined in this book: they eat nutrient-dense and minimally processed food, movement is part of their daily ritual, they have a strong community, they use their brains, they have purpose and they spend time outdoors. The Haenyeo, a group of female divers who reside on Jeju Island, off the south coast of South Korea, include women aged seventy and even older. This community of women harvests seafood by diving up to 10 metres into the sea without diving equipment or breathing apparatuses. These women represent what true health and longevity means to me – a strong female community, eating food from nature, spending more time outdoors, moving daily, having a sense of purpose – and in their case, even cold-water swimming and breathwork. This is how I want to age.

And this is why I often find the wellness industry so off-track with the fundamentals. How much simpler things would be if nourishing food, purpose and movement were just part of our routine. True health really depends on remembering the basics:

- We need to eat nourishing food.
- We need sunlight.
- We need fresh air.
- We need to follow the seasons.
- We need to sleep.
- We need to move.
- We need community.
- We need purpose.
- We need to have fun!

I see ageing as a journey towards wisdom, greater intuition and enrichment (or as close to that as we can get amid the day-to-day grind!). When I lived in Vietnam and China, older women – the matriarchs of the family – were revered, listened to and, to be honest, were the ones who really ran things. This contrasts with the attitude towards middle-aged women in the West, where we often feel invisible in society or even ridiculed (the expression 'a women of a certain age' springs to mind). In Traditional Chinese Medicine (which is around 5,000 years old) there is the term Second Spring, which refers to a positive reframing of post-menopause – a time of renewed vitality and opportunity. Menopause is a time of huge hormonal flux – our winter cycle in TCM requires us to withdraw before emerging into our Second Spring with new vigour and thoughts of new possibilities.

SECOND SPRING: THE LIBERATION AFTER MENOPAUSE

Kate Codrington
Author, speaker, artist

There is an awakening happening through perimenopause which can be hard to discern through the toxic fog of ageism and panic. Nevertheless, perimenopause has your back; she is bringing your attention to the beauty of your uniquely precious essence and preparing you for a Second Spring where you are ready to bring your unique gifts and skills to the world.

For centuries, we've been told that the end of menstruation is the end of purpose, sexuality and womanhood. That we should either back off as a raddled hag or fill our faces full of plastic in an attempt to retain the male gaze. In fact, the reverse is true. The biggest gift of menopause is that we no longer care what others think, we simply no longer give a fuck. This release allows us to follow the threads of our Calling, to make choices about sexuality that centre our pleasure, and to define for ourselves what version of 'woman' we would like to embody. Not to please, or conform, but for our own satisfaction.

To understand why it's such a powerful time, we need to decode the map we've been carrying in our bodies all along: the menstrual cycle. Ecofeminism has long recognized the relationship between women's bodies and the earth: our expansion and contraction, the inner tides building and releasing. While our culture worships constant productivity, and consistent output, female bodies offer a different story.

Throughout our menstruating years, if we are not on hormonal contraception, our energy rises and falls through our cycle. It builds from the end of menstruation to ovulation, when, buoyed by oestrogen, we reach outward with capacity and connection. After ovulation, energy turns inward. Progesterone calms the system and we become more sensitive, reflective, discerning. It is a deeply intelligent pattern: outward contribution balanced by inward restoration.

Each season of the cycle has gifts: Spring offers post-period hope. Summer, ovulatory joy and collaboration. Autumn gives premenstrual clarity and honesty. Winter, menstrual rest and deep intuition. Understood in this way, the menstrual cycle gives us access to more of ourselves while preventing burnout. If only we'd been taught this at puberty, imagine how different our lives would have been.

These seasons also map onto our lives, with a teen Spring full of curiosity as we find out who we are. A Life Summer of capacity and validation. A perimenopausal Life Autumn bringing sensitivity and seeing the truth, followed by a Life Winter of dreamy intuition.

We've spent the first half of our lives learning how to navigate a female-unfriendly world, weighing up appearance over comfort, juggling income with well-being, desire for a family with work. It is a long apprenticeship in bending ourselves into the required shape. Luckily, in these Summer years we have the capacity to be all things to all the people, and with oestrogen on our side, we are able to smile while we do them. The sensitive perimenopause years act as an Autumnal and Wintery season that invites us to step back from the world and let go of what is not serving us, to attend to life laundry, to our wounds and trauma. The Change is a change for the better.

Perimenopause is messy and confronting, yes. It needs to be to help us shake off the conditioning! It asks us to shed illusions, face betrayals, feel the griefs we've stuffed in the cupboard marked 'for later'. It strips us down to essence and insists we stop performing our way through the world. Deep, radical Wintery rest, nourishment, slowing down become requirements and, like all Winters, if we manage to meet it with even a spoonful of softness, a vibrant new season follows: Second Spring.

Just like our teen Spring, this early postmenopausal phase invites us to explore how to live with vibrancy in this older body. We step out of the menopause cave blinking, wobbly, while also carrying a profoundly strengthened sense of self. This is Second Spring: a time of curiosity, experimentation, new beginnings. In the second part of life, post-menopause, our Calling starts to speak to us loudly and this requires us to *not fit in*. In fact, to become more uniquely ourselves; more nerdy, more niche in our interests and pursuits. It's a time of expansion not driven by oestrogen, but by our inner authority. We get to try things on again to see how they feel: clothes, work, relationships, ways of expressing ourselves. We will inevitably overreach, fail, fall flat, our energy crash, and then return to the rest and nourishment we learned to honour during menopause. All the Autumnal and Wintery lessons from perimenopause and from the premenstrual phases are still in play.

The seasonal and lunar maps become newly relevant in Second Spring, guiding our energy though our new lives. Without the menstrual cycle to pace us, the body naturally seeks other rhythms. Some find themselves tuning into the moon, feeling energy rise at waxing, intensity at full, more sensitivity at waning, and needing rest at dark moon. Others find themselves aligning with the annual seasons, dreaming and visioning in winter, planting ideas in spring, full expression in summer, harvesting and simplifying in autumn. Our bodies don't lose cyclicity post-menopause; but reaching the calmer, quieter post-hormonal waters, they simply shift cycles.

Beyond Second Spring, the rest of the Second Cycle unfolds with its own richness. Second Summer in our sixties brings mastery and expansion of our Calling as we understand it. Second Autumn in our later years invites radical letting go, forgiveness and deep compassion. Second Winter, when it comes, asks us to ready ourselves for the greatest transition of all.

When we come to the end of menopause and enter Second Spring, we're shown that the end of one cycle is simply the beginning of a wilder, deeper, more sovereign one: at last **we stop being defined by the world and start making the world our own.**

Post-menopause we can strive to be the healthiest and happiest that we've ever been, once we start to look after ourselves more, start to nourish ourselves more and put ourselves at the top of that never-ending to-do list. I hope my advice will create abundant energy for you, so you can get on with all the things YOU want to do – which is far more important than focusing on your age and letting it dictate what you can and can't do. As I often say, our body is not a project. The project is to enjoy what it can do for you! I hope this book will furnish you with the ancient wisdom (and the scientific evidence, if you are interested in that side of things) to help maintain your strength, heart health, cognitive function and overall vitality post-menopause so that you can embrace your next chapter and future-proof your body at the same time, without the need for biohacks, expensive equipment or complicated protocols.

Let's build a life where nourishing food, purpose and movement are part of our routine and then longevity becomes a side effect rather than a goal.

post-menopause

AS THE GATEWAY TO OPTIMAL AGEING

I see menopause as a time of change when our body is often screaming at us to start looking after ourselves more, and that is why I view this transition as 'the gateway to optimal ageing'. The Office for National Statistics now tracks health span as well as life expectancy, which, in the UK, is 78.8 years for males and 82.8 years for females.[1] The UK Healthy Life Expectancy (health span) statistics are based on how an individual perceives their general health and has been estimated for males in England to be 61.5 years and 61.9 years for females.[2] That means the difference between how long you feel healthy versus your lifespan is 17 years for men and over 20 years for women! So, we might be living longer, but we live in poorer health for longer. However, we can change this. New research suggests that sustainable health gains for those who optimize their diet from age 20 can increase their life expectancy by up to a decade, and even at 60, it was estimated that you could still extend life expectancy by up to 8 years for women and 8.8 years for men.[3] Menopause is the health wake-up call we needed – it was worth it, I promise!

the hallmarks of ageing

Environmental factors, such as diet, stress, pollution, lifestyle (epigenetics) and genetics, play important roles in ageing. Studies have found that genes may be responsible for just 20 to 30 per cent of how we age.[4] The biochemical science of ageing is complex, but I shall aim to summarize it. The hallmarks of ageing are a group of biological traits agreed by the scientific community. There were nine areas included when they were first published in 2013 in the journal *Cell*: genomic instability, telomere attrition (shortening), epigenetic alterations, loss of proteostasis (protein balance), deregulated nutrient-sensing, mitochondrial dysfunction, cellular senescence (where cells stop dividing but don't die), stem cell exhaustion and altered intercellular communication. In 2023, three more were added: chronic inflammation, dysbiosis (an imbalance in the gut microbiome) and disabled macroautophagy (the ability of cells to self-clean and get rid of damaged components).[5] The inclusion of chronic inflammation and dysbiosis are interesting – as a nutritionist these are two areas I see a lot of in my clinic, considering that menopause is now viewed as an inflammatory transitional event in a woman's life due to oestrogen's role in the immune system.[6]

key ageing genes

The FOXO3 gene is often referred to as the 'longevity gene' because it's consistently associated with healthy ageing and longevity.[7] This gene is linked to insulin sensitivity, better physical and cognitive function in older age, and reduced DNA damage and cardiovascular disease, contributing to a longer health span and lifespan. FOXO3 has advantageous roles in the cell nucleus: it breaks down molecules called reactive oxygen species (ROS), and it helps regulate cell death, DNA repair, stem cell homeostasis and immune system modulation. FOXO3, along with another gene, NRF2, helps switch on the body's antioxidant protection system. Antioxidants help protect us from chronic conditions such as diabetes, cardiovascular disease, cancer and neurological disorders. Remember, our genes are important, but our environment is just as important because it affects how these genes are expressed. For example, antioxidants from our diet have been shown to increase FOXO3 activity. They include curcumin in turmeric, green tea catechins, resveratrol (found in grapes and red wine), astaxanthin (found in anything pink, such as salmon or prawns) and beta-hydroxybutyric acid, induced by fasting or exercise. But more on these later. Vitamin D, the sunshine vitamin, helps to slow down another gene, PARP1. Hyperfunction of this gene can lead to DNA repair errors and damage to cells, which is why being outside is so important for our health (in addition to supplementation all year round). The more we age, the more our FOXO3 expression can fluctuate, so we need to support it more, especially as the FOXO3 gene is expressed with the help of oestrogen – one of the reasons why women live longer than men, maybe?

Now on to SIRT genes. There are seven of these, responsible for the production of seven different sirtuins – proteins essential for the survival of all living cells. SIRT1 and SIRT3 are consistently linked to extended health span and longevity. They both activate FOXO3, regulate DNA repair and support cell survival and anti-inflammatory pathways. Sirtuins prevent cellular senescence (when cells stop dividing and can build up as we age), support cell survival, DNA repair, cell metabolism and cell proliferation, which is why their dysfunction is associated with age-related conditions such as cardiovascular disease, obesity, neurodegeneration and cancer. Sirtuin activity increases in a fasted state. Sirtuins are dependent on NAD+, a derivative of vitamin B3 (which is why there is so much noise around NAD+ injections) and polyphenols, such as quercetin (found in onions, leeks, apples and grapes), catechins from green tea, berberine (mainly in barberries, medicinal herbs and supplements), and resveratrol (in red grapes, red wine, blueberries, peanuts and dark chocolate).[8] As a nutritional therapist, NAD+ injections don't sit easy with me; I prefer to support the body's natural processes, in this case supporting NAD+ production, rather than giving high amounts of the end product, which might overstimulate certain functions. There is no quick fix to ageing well! We are very good at recycling B3 (niacin) to provide NAD+, although these pathways can slow as we age, so I do get why there is a market for these products. Foods high in B3 include liver, chicken breast (one fillet will give you over 80 per cent of your RDA), turkey, salmon, pulses, anchovies (just ten can provide over 50 per cent of your RDA), peanuts, avocados and brown rice. Green beans, tofu and edamame beans are high in nicotinamide mononucleotide (NMN), which is a direct precursor to NAD+. Exercise and a fasted state also stimulate NAD+.

supporting gene stability

Genomic instability is one of the hallmarks of ageing. Methylation is a mechanism behind the regulation of epigenetic gene expression (resulting from lifestyle factors). It is a key chemical process happening billions of times every second in virtually every cell in the body, constantly and dynamically regulating our daily functions. A particular kind of methylation, DNA methylation, is where a methyl group is added to a DNA molecule, which can turn genes 'off' or silence them without changing the DNA sequence itself. It acts a bit like a dimmer switch. Ageing is closely linked to changes in DNA methylation. Methylation underpins many key processes in the body, for example: DNA methylation (synthesis and repair), homocysteine recycling (a big factor when it comes to our cardiovascular health – we don't want high homocysteine levels), pregnancy, hormone balance and neurotransmitter synthesis (including the on/off switch that controls them). Methylation also supports the production of an important antioxidant called glutathione, which helps reduce inflammation, supports detoxification, helps repair oxidative stress, and prevents neurological damage and autoimmunity from developing.

Dietary folate (vitamin B9) is hugely important for methylation. It is found in abundance in green leafy vegetables (spinach, kale, watercress), which is why they are such an important part of our diet post-menopause. Other sources include lentils, beans, peas, chickpeas, sunflower seeds, hazelnuts and liver. Folate is different from folic acid, the latter being the man-made form of vitamin B9, which can be much harder for those with a particular genetic variance to metabolize. This is why I always recommend the folate form from food and in supplements. Like folate, B12 is also important to support methylation, which is why low folate and B12 impact this process. Methylation is also supported by choline (eggs are a great source), B vitamins (in particular B1, B3, B6, B9 – folate – and B12), zinc, potassium and magnesium, omega-3 DHA, and the amino acids methionine, cysteine and taurine. Polyphenols (see pp.25–6) are also incredibly important as they help to promote balanced DNA methylation and include turmeric, EGCG from green tea, rosmarinic acid (rosemary), lycopene (tomatoes), genistein (soy), quercetin (apples, grapes, onions, capers, broccoli) and vitamins A, C and D. It's also important to avoid 'damage amplifiers' such as high blood sugar, high alcohol consumption, smoking, charred meats, ultra-processed foods and xenoestrogens (synthetic chemicals that mimic oestrogen and can be hormone disruptors).

telomere shortening

Telomere shortening (attrition) is another hallmark of ageing. Telomeres are the protective caps that sit on top of the very ends of each of our chromosomes. The length of our telomeres is considered to be one of the best markers of biological age, and there are now over-the-counter blood tests available for this, although they can be prohibitively expensive. If telomeres shorten too much, our cells can no longer divide and they become 'senescent', which basically means they become worn out and are unable to replicate. These now obsolete cells can build up and increase inflammation in the body, although a well-functioning immune system can detect and clear these damaged cells (in a process known as autophagy). So how do we stop our telomeres from shortening too rapidly? By eating a nutrient-rich diet full of antioxidants and omega-3s, which help protect telomeres from damage, as well as exercising and reducing the intake of ultra-processed foods.

autophagy

Disabled autophagy is one of the hallmarks of ageing. It is one kind of a process called autophagy. This is the general term for the body's way of cleaning and recycling damaged or old parts inside cells. Macroautophagy is the main way the clean-up gets done – where the cell wraps up waste and breaks it down for reuse. It's an essential part of keeping cells healthy, and the great news is, there are many ways our diet and lifestyle can support this process. We can induce autophagy with exercise, EGCG from green tea, extra virgin olive oil, thyme and oregano. Longer overnight fasting can also restore autophagy signalling.[9]

'inflamm-ageing'

As mentioned earlier, chronic inflammation was added to the hallmarks of ageing in 2023 and it is deeply interconnected with a process called epigenetics – the way that lifestyle factors affect our genes and how we age. As you will see, there is an inflammatory component to all the health concerns I discuss in this book. Inflammation can negatively affect DNA repair, alter cell signalling, gut dysbiosis and telomere shortening.[10] Oestrogen functions as an anti-inflammatory agent, so this is why, during menopause, as levels drop, we can suffer with more pro-inflammatory symptoms, such as aches and pains, bloating, gum disease, eczema and other inflammatory skin issues. Getting inflammation under control is therefore central to our health post-menopause.

When the process is in balance, inflammation increases free radical production. Our immune cells are part of the inflammatory response, producing large amounts of reactive oxygen species (ROS) – free radicals – to help fight pathogens. We also produce free radicals during metabolism and detoxification, as well as in response to pollution, low-nutrient diets, stress and smoking. However, when the immune system is out of balance, chronic inflammation occurs, which leads to more free radicals. Free radicals are unstable molecules that can damage cells, leading to more inflammation and oxidative stress. An inflammatory catch-22 ensues. A simple analogy for oxidation is when you cut an apple and see it go brown and start to rot. Exactly the same process takes place in human cells. Antioxidants are really important because they neutralize free radicals, slowing down or preventing oxidation. An out-of-balance antioxidant-to-free radical ratio leads to oxidative stress, which can lead to chronic disease. Cholesterol is not harmful until it is oxidized within the arterial walls. This oxidation process can be a key factor in the onset of atherosclerosis, or hardening of the arteries. The body does produce its own powerful antioxidants including glutathione, superoxide dismutase and catalase, but we also need to get antioxidants from the food that we eat – from vitamins C and E as well as minerals that are crucial for the body's own antioxidant enzymes to work properly. These include selenium, zinc and manganese, and polyphenols, which have potent antioxidant roles in the body. This is why an antioxidant-rich diet is crucial post-menopause, to help protect us from cellular damage and reduce the impact of oxidative stress to slow biological ageing and reduce inflammation.

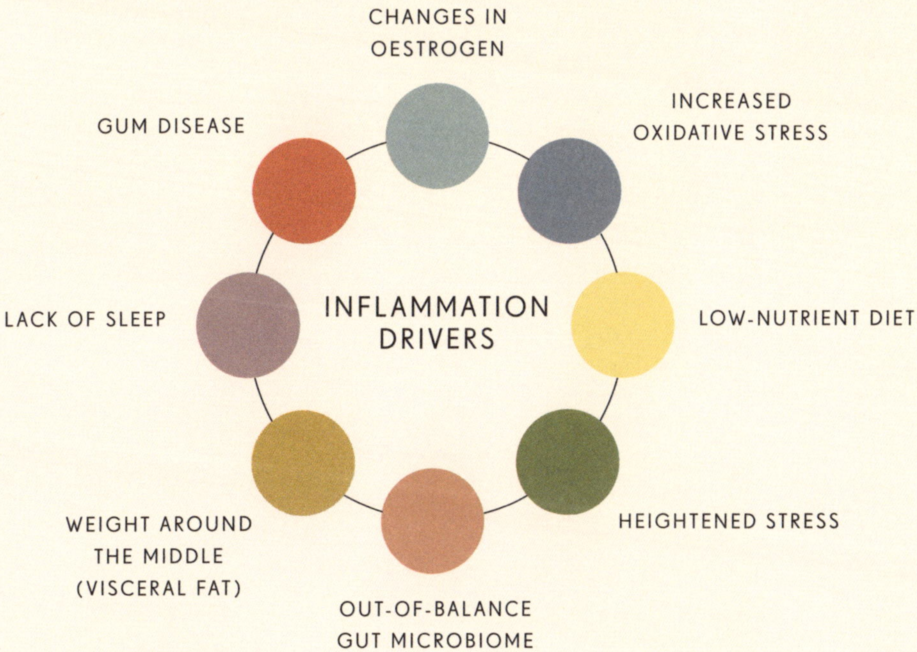

mitochondrial health – our energy factories

Mitochondrial dysfunction is yet another of the hallmarks of ageing and can often cause symptoms such as low energy, brain fog and issues with our ability to be metabolically flexible (see more in the Metabolic Harmony chapter). Mitochondria are the cells' energy factories. We have mitochondria in most of our cells (although none in red blood cells), with anything from 100 to 1,000 found in most cells, although power-hungry cells such as those found in the liver have around 1,000 to 2,000, heart cells have 5,000 to 8,000, and a large neuron (brain cell) can have over 1 million, and some have over 2 million! Mitochondria take carbohydrates, fats and, when these are in short supply, amino acids (these are not the preferred source), along with oxygen and convert them into the body's main energy currency – ATP. Your cells then use ATP to power everything from thinking and moving to repairing and healing. Mitochondria produce high levels of free radicals due to this metabolism, which the body needs to mop up with antioxidants. Polyphenols are crucial, especially sage, curcumin, rosemary, quercetin, resveratrol and EGCG from green tea – more on these later. The omega-3 fatty acid DHA (found in oily fish, or broken down from plant-based omega-3 sources such as linseed/flaxseed oil), the omega-6 fatty acid linoleic acid (found in nuts and seeds) and extra virgin olive oil are particularly important for the integrity of the inner mitochondrial membrane. Cold water exposure can support the ETC and heat stress (saunas) can also support mitochondrial balance. Time-restricted eating and exercise are important for our mitochondrial health too, along with key nutrients: magnesium, zinc, selenium, B vitamins, vitamin D and E, CoQ10 and iron.[11]

Over the next few pages, I will cover some of the dietary highlights that underpin the Post-Menopause Method.

nutrient density

Nutrient density is key to improving biomarkers related to high cholesterol, blood sugar, inflammation, oxidative stress, and immune function. I have collated my top eighteen health span-enhancing ingredients into what I have named the Longevity Larder, which you will encounter in the next chapter and see referenced throughout this book.

When it comes to dietary patterns and the hallmarks of ageing, the Mediterranean diet has been the most researched and has been shown to provide huge benefits across all hallmarks. It is rich in plant-based foods such as vegetables, fruit, legumes, grains, nuts and seeds, along with high intakes of fish. Red meat, ultra-processed foods and dairy products are eaten less frequently. It is also very high in vitamins and minerals, fibre, monounsaturated (from extra virgin olive oil) and polyunsaturated fats (from the oily fish) and polyphenols, which don't come up in any RDA list, but should, in my opinion (see pp.25–6). I would also like to add that many diets around the world also include many of the same dietary elements, bar perhaps the olive oil. The Mediterranean diet has been shown to positively support all of the hallmarks of ageing.[12] It is associated with longer telomeres along with lower inflammation,[13] and it first attracted researchers because of better cardiovascular-disease outcomes in the region. Higher adherence to the Mediterranean diet was associated with reduced risks of chronic diseases including cardiovascular disease,[14] type 2 diabetes,[15] neurodegenerative disease[16] and cancer. The Mediterranean diet also includes many elements that have been shown to have positive effects on promoting DNA repair, which can be affected by ageing, such as glucosinolates in cruciferous vegetables (broccoli, cabbage, kale, cavolo nero and sprouts), nuts such as walnuts,[17] extra virgin olive oil[18] (even tomato sauce cooked with olive oil demonstrates this protective effect), spinach and blueberries.

The Blue Zones are places in the world noted for their high numbers of centenarians and reduced instances of diabetes and cardiovascular disease. They don't share the same diet, but they have patterns of eating in common. Food is seasonal and high in antioxidants: purple sweet potato and soya in Okinawa; tomatoes, nuts, seeds and olive oil in Sardinia and Ikaria, Greece; corn, squash, beetroot, papaya and black beans in Nicoya, Costa Rica. Their diets are also high in plants, and high in pulses – Nicoyans eat beans daily, while in the UK we struggle with half a portion a week, and that usually comes from ultra-processed baked beans. Their diets are high in fibre, which supports their microdiversity, and fermentation is used to extend the harvest and benefit from the live bacteria (found in the sourdough bread and soft cheese common to Sardinia). Their diets are high in polyphenols, too, known to support the FOXO3 gene – the curcumin and catechins (from green tea) common in the Okinawans' diet may in part explain their longevity. Although canned spam was introduced to Okinawa by the US Army at the end of World War 2, they are now one of the world's largest consumers of it! I shan't be recommending that! All Blue Zones consume a lot of soups and fish, but meat is a side dish rather than the main event. Many of the Blue Zones are islands, too, often with different food cultures to their mainlands, and they often eat what they can grow locally. Inhabitants have a lot of stress resilience as they often live in close-knit, rural communities, and older people are much more active. Here, there is no need to go the gym as people are often gardening or walking up steep inclines. They don't snack either, and adhere to semi time-restricted eating, reflecting the Japanese expression *hara hachi bu*, eating until you are 80 per cent full.

There is also much we can learn from the health outcomes in countries that have some of the oldest humans on earth, such as in Japan, where the diet is also full of plants, oily fish, wholegrains, seeds (fewer nuts though) and minimal meat (meat makes up around 1 per cent of the Okinawan diet[19]), sugar and ultra-processed foods. They also have the added advantage of more phytoestrogen-rich soy in their diet, which is incredibly helpful for us at menopause[20] and which is harder to incorporate into Mediterranean-style cooking. They also engage in what is known as 'social nutrition', where food is eaten with friends and family and constitutes an important part of their daily life. It is not to be rushed or eaten in front of screens, or skipped or eaten on the go, like most of us often do. (More on these longevity lifestyle patterns later.)

polyphenols

Aside from vitamins, minerals, fibre and mono- and polyunsaturated fats, polyphenols are among the most important elements of a nutrient-dense diet designed to promote our post-menopausal health. Diets rich in polyphenols are associated with an extended health span because they interact with many of the hallmarks of ageing. Polyphenols are plant chemicals found in large amounts in brightly coloured fruits and vegetables, extra virgin olive oil, tea, coffee, herbs, spices and pulses, and they exert super-important qualities when it comes to inflammation and ageing. Many polyphenols are powerful antioxidants, which help to reduce inflammation and the risk of systemic conditions such as cardiovascular disease, diabetes and obesity. Antioxidants help to protect our cells from damage caused by free radicals, which are unstable molecules that can lead to cell and DNA damage. Polyphenols help to protect plants from disease, and as such, help us too! In nature, stress drives resilience. The more stress the plant is under, the more polyphenols it creates for protection. This is why organic ginger, for example, will taste more fiery than normal ginger – organic farming does not use pesticides or herbicides, so the ginger needs to create greater quantities of gingerols to protect itself against pests.[21] Olive trees, which grow in very harsh, arid environments, are known to produce greater amounts of polyphenols.[22] Polyphenols are split into four main families: flavonoids, which is the largest (with subcategories including quercetin, catechins, flavones and anthocyanins); phenolic acids; stilbenes (such as resveratrol); and lignans (found in ground linseed/flaxseed, sesame seeds, brassicas, peppers, French beans, carrots and cashews). Polyphenols have a powerful antioxidant, antimicrobial, anti-inflammatory and antihypertensive action, which is hugely beneficial for our health span.[23] They are also hugely beneficial for our gut health, which is where two thirds of our immune system resides. Studies suggest that they can help to reduce inflammation and support gut integrity,[24] and also slow down telomere shortening.[25] Polyphenols have also been shown to support our cells' energy factories – the mitochondria. Ageing can reduce the efficiency of our mitochondria, reducing energy levels and increasing free radicals, which can lead to more oxidative stress. This can then lead to mitochondrial dysfunction (as discussed on p.22). Polyphenols such as resveratrol, curcumin, hydroxytyrosol and oleuropein (found in olive oil) have been shown to stimulate mechanisms involved in supporting mitochondrial balance.

So here are some examples of polyphenols that are often present in scientific research (over 8,000 varieties have been identified), which will pop up again in later chapters, alongside the ingredients that contain high amounts of them. These need to be added to your shopping list!

- Anthocyanins: found in acai berries, elderberries, blackcurrants, red cabbage, purple sweet potatoes, cacao and blueberries
- Apigenin: in grapefruit, parsley, onions, oranges, tea and celery
- Catechins: in tea (esepcially green tea and matcha), cacao and dark chocolate, apples, blackberries and cherries
- Chlorogenic acid: mostly found in coffee beans
- Curcumin: found in turmeric
- Ellagic acid: in berries, pomegranates, walnuts and pecans
- Epigallocatechin gallate (EGCG): in green tea and matcha
- Gallic acid: in berries, pineapples, bananas and lemons
- Genistein: in soybeans and soy-derived foods such as tofu, tempeh, edamame beans and miso, as well as broad beans
- Gingerols: found in ginger
- Hydroxytyrosol: primarily found in extra virgin olive oil
- Kaempferol: a flavanoid found in kale, broccoli, tea, grapes, beans and tomatoes
- Lignans: in ground linseed/flaxseed, sesame seeds and red alfafa
- Oleuropein: found in extra virgin olive oil
- Procyanidins: found in apples, dark chocolate and grapes
- Quercetin: in onions, broccoli, apples, apricots, berries, nuts, seeds, tea, wine and cacao/dark chocolate
- Resveratrol: found in red grape skin, red wine, berries and peanuts
- Rosmarinic acid: in herbs, especially rosemary, mint and lemon balm
- Sesamin: a lignan polyphenol found in sesame seeds

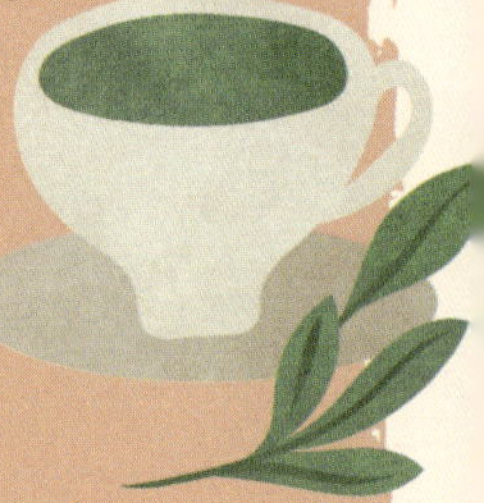

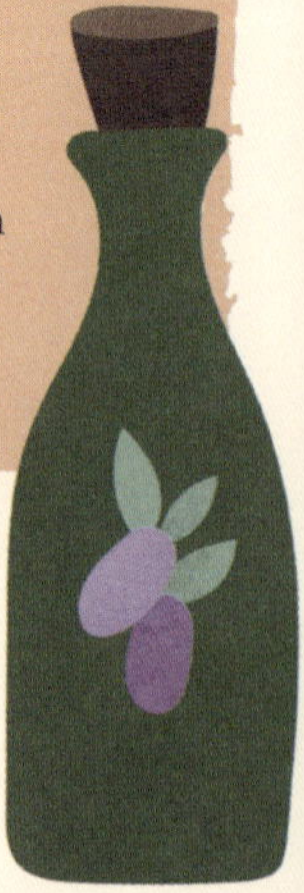

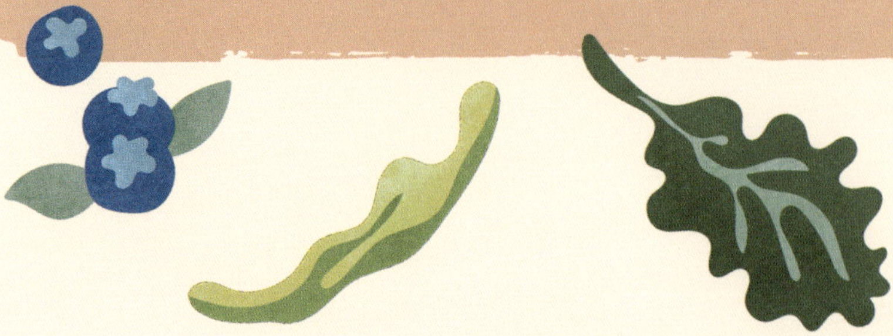

fibre

One of the biggest advantages of the Mediterranean style of eating, and the core component that we see across the world in regions with some of the healthiest and longest-living women (and men!), is a high intake of plants. And this means a high intake of fibre. It still staggers me that in the UK, 90 per cent of us are still not getting the recommended daily 30 grams of fibre. Beans are central to the Blue Zones diets and are affordable, versatile (many of my recipes contain them), and one of the most studied, evidence-backed foods in nutritional science. Higher legume intake is consistently linked with better blood-sugar control, lower stroke risk and better metabolic health. Half a cup delivers 8 to 11 grams of protein, plus fibre, B vitamins, iron, magnesium, antioxidants and no cholesterol. If you eat a diet high in plants for breakfast, lunch and dinner, you will smash this target, and both my *Natural Menopause Method Cookbook*, and the additional recipes here, will help you reach it.

In an analysis of a large European prospective study of over 450,000 men and women, a higher fibre intake was shown to be associated with lower mortality, particularly from circulatory, digestive and non-cardiovascular, non-cancer inflammatory diseases.[26] Even increasing fibre intake by just 8 to 10 grams a day has been shown to result in a 15 to 30 per cent decrease in all-cause and cardiovascular-related mortality when comparing people who eat the highest amount of fibre to those who eat the least.[27] The study of the microbiome in centenarians and other elderly people has revealed how changes in diversity can cause inflammation, which can lead to an increase in age-related disease, which is why gut dysbiosis is one of the hallmarks of ageing. Gut dysbiosis can lead to gut permeability, the accumulation of pro-inflammatory commensals (bacteria that live in our gut but have to be kept in check) and the reduction of beneficial microbes. Gut microbes in super-agers still show an abundance of beneficial bacteria, especially *Akkermansia muciniphila*, which helps to support gut-wall integrity and gut microbe diversity.[28] A prolonged lack of fibre can affect these important microbes.[29]

fasting

One of the original hallmarks of ageing listed back in 2013 was deregulated nutrient-sensing. Research has suggested that fasting, and therefore reducing the stimulation of nutrients that comes with eating, can encourage the cell repair process. In Ikaria, Greece, one of the Blue Zones, fasting is part of the Greek Orthodox religion, requiring people to fast on Wednesdays and Fridays. This means no meat, fish, eggs or dairy – legumes are allowed (especially chickpeas and lentils). Research has found that calorie reduction can support autophagy (the body's way of cleaning and recycling damaged or old parts inside cells) and might reduce inflammation.

New research on chrononutrition, the study of when we eat, may shape how our organs age.[30] A recent study of 14,000+ adults found that different organs age at different rates and that our meal timings might relate to biological ageing. Eating the last meal before 9pm was associated with slower ageing of the body, particularly the heart and liver. Eating between 3–5pm was associated with body and heart support, and from 5 to 7pm, liver support. Signs of accelerated biological ageing were associated with late first meals (skipping breakfast!) and longer eating windows of more than 8 hours a day. The effects were more marked in adults over 40 – particularly in men, and in people with pre-existing health conditions, so this has to be taken into account, but it certainly reflects my approach from a nutritional-therapy perspective: meal timing and reduced eating windows may be just as important as what we are eating when it comes to healthy ageing.

A really simple way to start fasting today is to eat your evening meal earlier than planned, then eat tomorrow's breakfast later. So, eat around 6 to 6:30pm if you can, and then don't eat your breakfast until 9am. I also recommend mini-fasts between meals, and if you do want something sweet like some dark chocolate after your evening meal (I do most nights!), then eat this soon after your meal.

stress adaptation

We must also factor into this the high life-load we are experiencing at midlife. The to-do lists, the stress, the lack of recovery – the constant tiger in the room, as I like to call it – all increase inflammation. Remember that our bodies have evolved over millennia and can't always tell the difference between needing to run from or fight a wild animal, and sitting at a desk getting stressed out over work, or panicking while stuck in a traffic jam. The biochemical reaction is the same. Constant stress (remember that busy can also equal stress) and other lifestyle factors, such as smoking, obesity, a sedentary lifestyle, poor sleep and pollution, can affect our telomere length and inflammation. Sadly, we can't go and live on a desert island, but we can help our bodies adapt to the stress that we encounter every day. My biggest bit of advice is to eat a protein-rich breakfast and to not skip meals (more of this in the Metabolic Harmony chapter), because balancing blood sugar levels is key to reducing stress hormones. Other areas to focus on include exercising to reduce anxiety (I exercise more for my mental health than my physical health a lot of the time!); reducing caffeine and alcohol, and only consuming them with food to reduce their effects; reducing sugar and ultra-processed foods; getting outside; cooking from scratch more (remember that 15 minutes is just 1 per cent of our day); eating more magnesium-rich foods (green leafy vegetables, avocadoes, cashews, pumpkin seeds and black beans); enjoying a magnesium salt bath before bed; and going to bed at a similar time every night. Adaptogens in supplement form can also be useful, such as ashwagandha, *Rhodiola rosea*, maca, cordyceps and *Panax ginseng* (Korean ginseng). If you suffer from a lot of anxiety, then lemon balm and L-theanine (found in green tea) can be helpful – green tea has been used for millenia for relaxation. You can also get these in supplement form: BioCare makes a good Calm Complex and Viridian makes a combined Lemon Balm and L-theanine supplement.

I know that was a lot of science, but I always think it is important to be mindful of the complexity of the body as an interconnected system. Yet it's also important for me to keep it simple so that you can make obtainable (not stress-inducing!) long-term nutritional shifts that will make you feel great immediately and help reduce your longer-term risk of chronic disease.

LET'S CELEBRATE BEING POST-MENOPAUSE

Professor Joyce Harper

Scientist, author and women's health educator

Women are being told that menopause is a terrible life stage and that when our periods stop, we will turn into dried up old crones. Guess what – it doesn't need to be this way. I look on post-menopause as a time of freedom and liberation: free from our menstrual cycle, free from fluctuating reproductive hormones (which can have a huge effect on our physical and mental health), free from periods, and free from the need for contraception. It can also be a time when women find their authentic self. It is often called The Change, and many women do change.

But we are ageing from the minute we are born, and there is no quick fix to ageing well. Menopause can be a wake-up call to look after our well-being through self-care. For me, lifestyle is the most important way we can support our good health and happiness. A healthy lifestyle is the best preventative medicine. Many research studies show that a healthy lifestyle reduces the risk of chronic health conditions, which becomes even more important as we age. These include dementia, Alzheimer's, obesity, cardiac and respiratory disorders, diabetes and cancer.

I feel so strongly about this that I interviewed 50 thriving women over 50 to share their wisdom, all covered in my latest book, *Your Joyful Years: Empowering Good Health and Happiness Beyond 50*. I asked them about the pillars of health: nutrition, exercise, sleep, mental health, and friendships and community, as well as the pillars of happiness – hobbies, creativity, time in nature, quality time alone, sex, a sense of purpose, and the wonders of travel, adventures and challenges.

If we want to age well, we need to make sure we have fun and joy in our lives. You may wonder why happiness matters for ageing well. Activities that bring us joy can reduce stress hormones such as cortisol and increase 'happy' hormones and neurotransmitters. These include dopamine, serotonin, oxytocin, endorphins, and our natural endocannabinoids. Together, they help lift mood; reduce stress; create feelings of pleasure, calm and connection; support better sleep and mental resilience; reduce inflammation; and strengthen immune, cardiovascular and metabolic function. Neuroscience studies suggest that activities such as exercise, meaningful social contact, time in nature and acts of kindness can increase the release of these chemicals and support our overall sense of well-being.

For some women, joy is rediscovering play: dancing, swimming outdoors, singing, drumming, painting, gardening, learning a language, joining a walking group, going to festivals, or travelling somewhere you've always wanted to go. For others it's smaller but just as meaningful: reading in peace, cooking with friends, sitting in a sauna, making time for a morning walk, or finding a hobby that absorbs you so completely you forget the clock. What matters is that it feels like yours.

Of course, not everyone experiences post-menopause as joyful. Some women have significant symptoms and health challenges and deserve care, treatment and compassion. Celebrating post-menopause should never mean dismissing those experiences. It's about widening the narrative so that women who are thriving feel seen, and women who are struggling know there are options and support.

One of the biggest barriers to ageing well is permission. Many women are brilliant at caring for everyone else and terrible at caring for themselves. We postpone our own needs because we're busy, because we feel guilty or because we've been taught that self-care is indulgent. But prioritizing self-care isn't selfish. It is maintenance. It is prevention. It is how we protect our health, our relationships and our capacity to enjoy our lives.

So let's do it. Let's make a deal with ourselves, and with each other. Let's stop talking about menopause as an ending and start talking about it as a new chapter – one with more freedom, more honesty and more fun. Let's build lives that include joy on purpose. Because ageing well isn't about trying to stay young. It's about being happy in the present.

the longevity larder

the top 18 ingredients for your capsule larder

The Longevity Larder is a capsule larder showcasing my top 18 ingredients, often imbedded in ancient patterns of eating. Modern-day nutritional science can now explain the mechanisms behind how they support our post-menopausal health and longevity. You will see these ingredients mentioned frequently throughout each chapter, with the most up-to-date research supporting their role in chronic disease prevention. All of the recipes have a Longevity Larder score, which gives a point for each ingredient used from the larder. This is where food becomes preventative medicine and the ultimate longevity 'biohack'.

1. EXTRA VIRGIN OLIVE OIL – POLYPHENOL POWERHOUSE

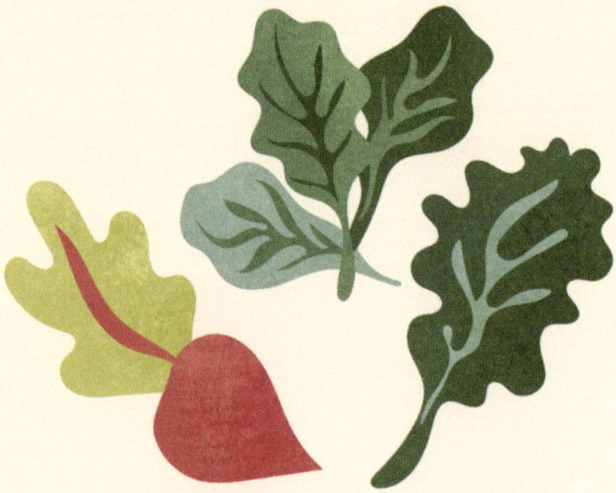

2. GREEN LEAFY VEGETABLES – POLYPHENOLS, VITAMINS, MINERALS & FIBRE

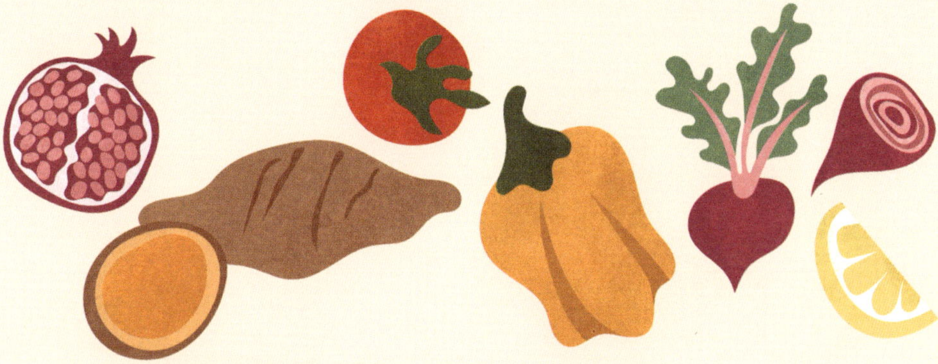

3. BRIGHTLY COLOURED (INCLUDING WHITE) FRUIT & VEG – ANTIOXIDANTS, POLYPHENOLS, VITAMINS & FIBRE

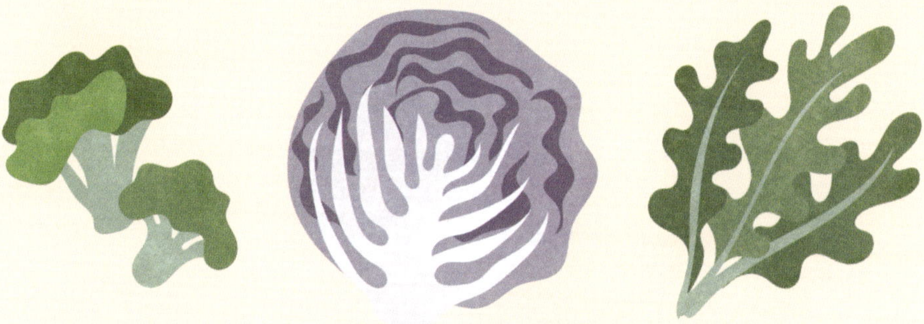

4. CRUCIFEROUS VEGETABLES – LIVER-LOVING GREENS

5. BERRIES & CHERRIES – POLYPHENOL POWERHOUSES & FIBRE

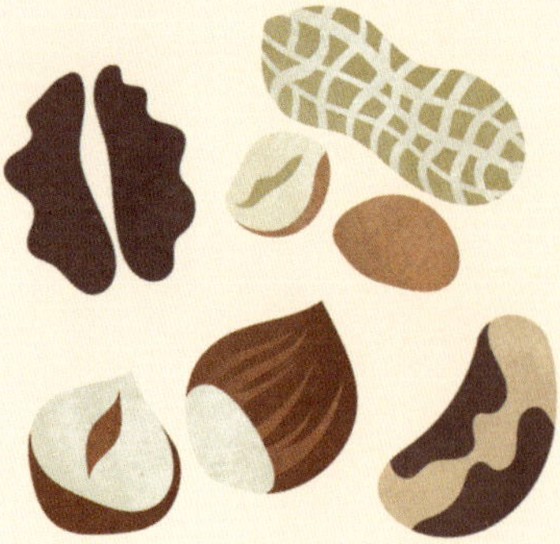

6. NUTS – ESSENTIAL FATTY ACIDS & POLYPHENOLS

7. SEEDS – PROTEIN, POLYPHENOLS & MINERALS

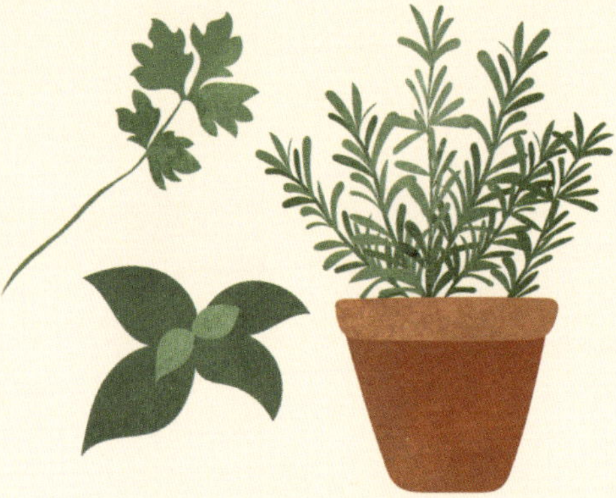

8. HERBS – POLYPHENOLS, VITAMINS & MINERALS

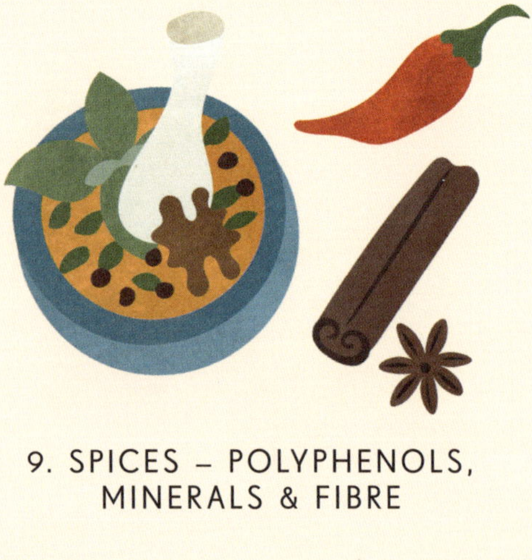

9. SPICES – POLYPHENOLS, MINERALS & FIBRE

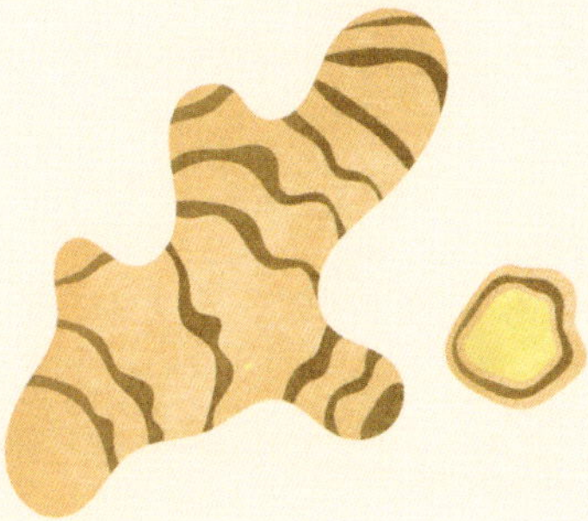

10. GINGER –
POLYPHENOLS,
ANTIOXIDANT &
ANTI-INFLAMMATORY

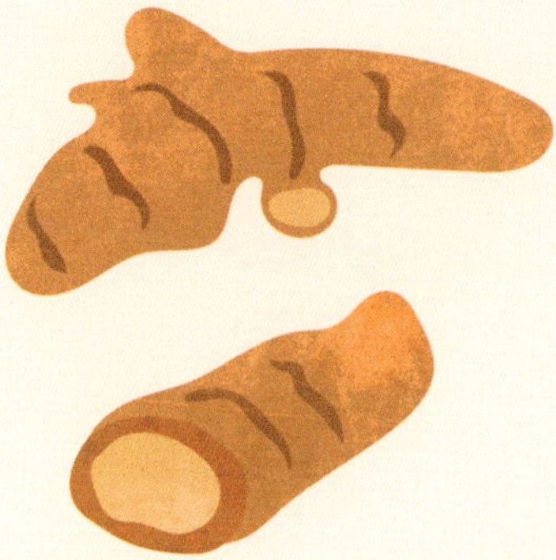

11. TURMERIC –
ANTI-INFLAMMATORY,
ANTIOXIDANT & LIVER-LOVING

12. GREEN TEA – CATECHIN
POLYPHENOL EGCG &
L-THEANINE

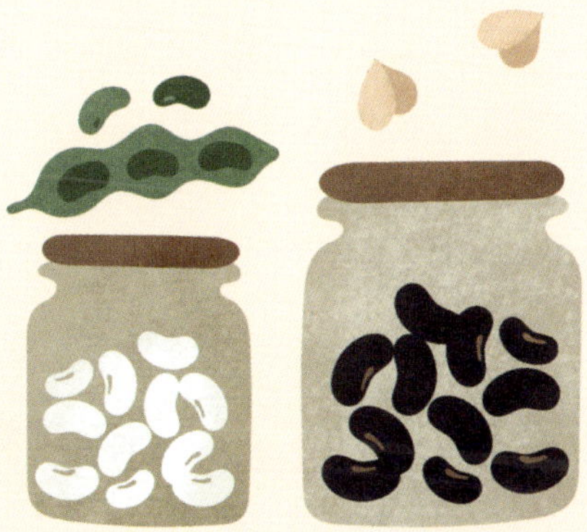

13. PULSES – FIBRE, PROTEIN
& PHYTOESTROGENS

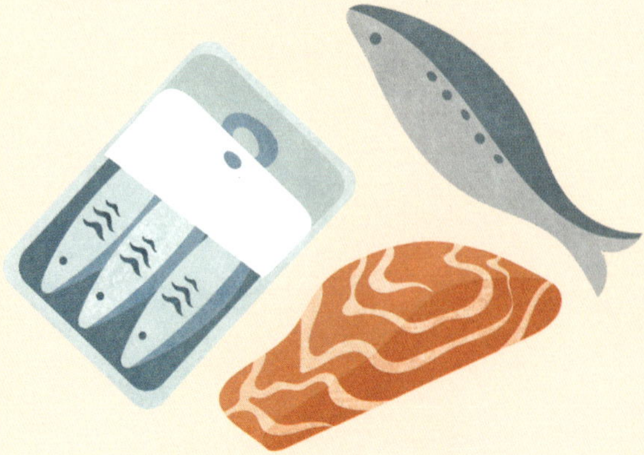

14. OILY FISH – OMEGA-3S
& ESSENTIAL AMINO ACIDS

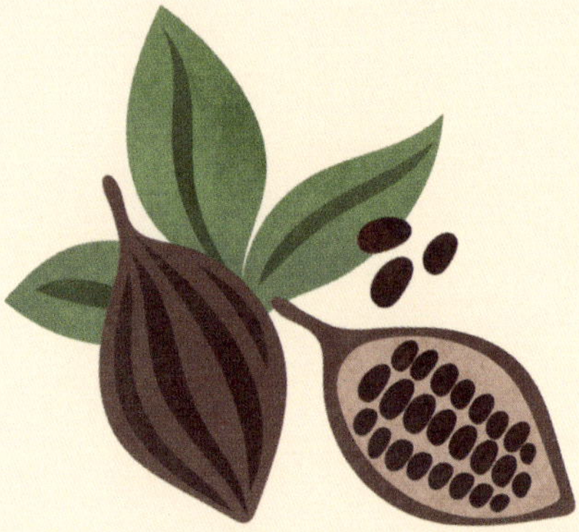

15. CACAO –
POLYPHENOL-RICH

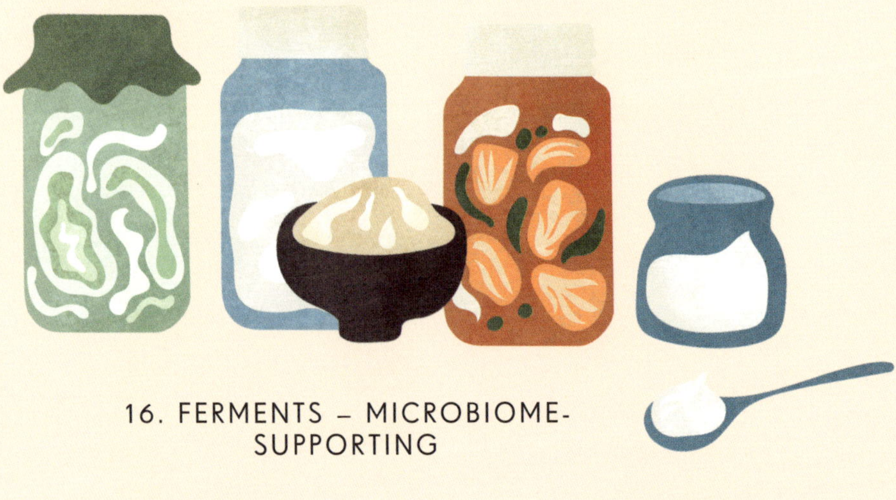

16. FERMENTS – MICROBIOME-
SUPPORTING

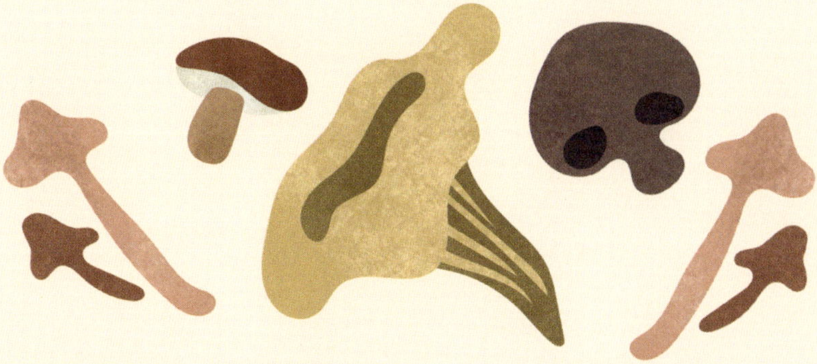

17. MUSHROOMS – POLYPHENOLS, GLUTATHIONE & ADAPTOGENS (FROM MEDICINAL MUSHROOMS)

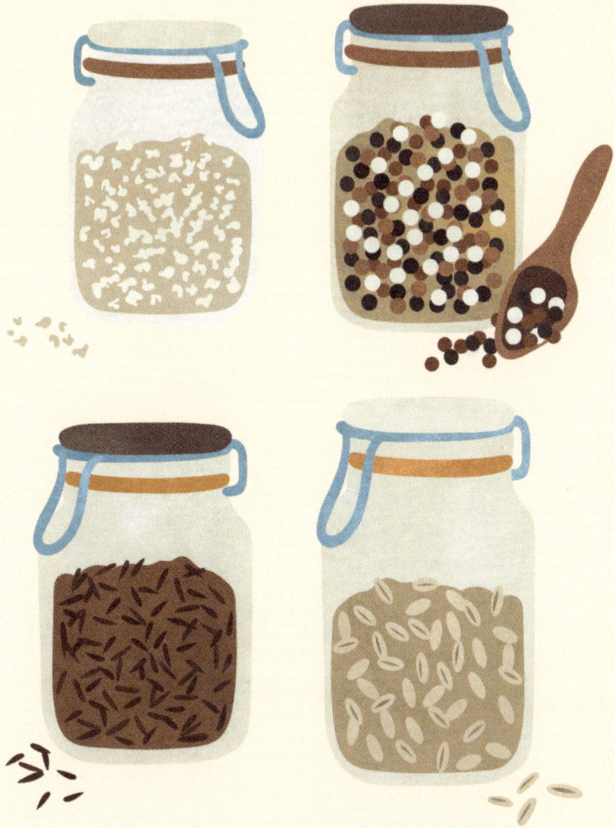

18. WHOLEGRAINS – MICROBIOME-SUPPORTING

metabolic harmony

Our post-menopausal metabolic health is so interconnected with our cardiovascular, brain, bone and immune health. Oestrogen is involved with many aspects of our metabolism: hunger and satiety cues, fat burning, glucose metabolism, glucose storage, insulin resistance and fat storage. Oestrogen regulates food intake by supporting leptin (our satiety hormone) and ghrelin (our hunger hormone). It can inhibit the hunger pathway, meaning that lower levels during post-menopause can result in more hunger signals. The fact that oestrogen supports leptin is one of the reasons why we often started to crave more food just before our period, when oestrogen was at its lowest. Post-menopause, low oestrogen can promote hunger, reduce satiety and lower energy expenditure. But we can gain back this balance – adaptation is key, and no strict diets!

how to stay metabolically healthy and flexible

Oestrogen is one of the many regulators of what are known as nutrient-sensing pathways, the mTOR and AMPK pathways. Dysfunction of nutrient-sensing is one of the hallmarks of ageing (see p.16). We don't want too much activation of one pathway – we want to have a balance, and to be able to switch between them smoothly. The mTOR pathway switches on when your body senses you are in a fed state, and the AMPK pathway switches on when your body is low in energy (for example, if you haven't eaten for a while, or if you're exercising). The mTOR pathway puts your body into growth and construction mode: cell division, tissue repair, and bone and muscle growth. These are the factors that upregulate it: protein intake, insulin, glucose, inflammatory messengers (cytokines), growth factors, excess calories, obesity, insulin resistance (thus higher insulin), a sedentary lifestyle, osteoporosis and visceral fat. The balancing AMPK pathway is upregulated in a fasted/calorie-restriction state (even a low blood-sugar state), which stimulates the body and brain to break down stored fat as ketones for energy. Other factors that can upregulate the AMPK pathway are extreme heat or cold, exercise, the diabetes drug metformin, and foods like chilli, quercetin-containing onions, leeks, apples and grapes, and EGCG, found in green tea. The key to metabolic health lies in our body's ability to switch between these pathways. Both are very important. We need growth post-menopause via the mTOR pathway, to build strong bones, muscle protein synthesis for lean muscle (for strength and fat loss) and for our immune system. But we also don't want to be in a constant fed state, which can lead to central weight gain and a quietening of the AMPK pathway. We need fasted periods and exercise to switch on the AMPK pathway for cellular repair and healthy fat burn too. Too much of the mTOR pathway (constant eating, lack of exercise) can lead to constant growth, which can lead to wear and tear over time. Too much of the AMPK pathway (constant restriction) means not enough bone and muscle building, and loss of strength. Our brain is super-sensitive to both these pathways. It needs to be able to switch to burning ketones when glucose is in short supply. This is central to brain adaptation post-menopause, as was highlighted in research by Dr Lisa Mosconi, Dr Roberta Brinton and their colleagues in 2021.[31]

Stress is a major driver of stubborn weight gain – I mean, who isn't stressed these days? And then menopause hits! Weight around the middle is also known as 'the worry waist', as our stress chemistry wants the body to hold onto fat ready for the next stress event; elevated cortisol promotes visceral fat due a perceived threat – the tiger in the room! As I mentioned before, the brain doesn't realize that we are getting stressed over spreadsheets – unfortunately, the biochemical responses are the same because this is an ancient survival reflex. This is why exercise is so important as a de-stressor (although over-exercising can be a stressor), as is making time in your busy day to cook because balancing your blood sugar will stop more of the stress response (see below). Adaptogens such as reishi mushrooms, cordyceps, *Rhodiola rosea*, ashwagandha and even turmeric can be helpful. These have been used for millennia in Ayurvedic and Traditional Chinese Medicine to blunt the cortisol response. Massage, acupuncture, magnesium salt baths, going to bed at the same time each night, reducing scrolling past 9pm, reading and seeing friends are also very important for our well-being.

oestrogen and blood sugar

Oestrogen fluctuations affect our ability to handle blood-sugar levels, which can have a knock-on effect on cravings, calorie intake, hanger, insulin resistance, high cholesterol and weight distribution around the middle. This is why our risk of insulin-resistant diabetes can increase post-menopause. Oestrogen helps to get glucose out of the blood and into our skeletal muscle cells, fat cells and liver cells, where it is stored as glycogen. It also aids a process called glycolysis, whereby glucose is burned to produce the body's energy currency, ATP. Low blood sugar can create more stress in the body as this results in the release of cortisol, adrenaline and noradrenaline (adrenaline and noradrenaline are part of the process of vasoconstriction, which increases blood pressure, and skin vasodilation, which can bring on hot flushes). This affects our brain, which doesn't like dips in blood sugar and responds by stimulating a stress cascade of chemicals to drive us to eat something sweet to get blood sugar back up again. Healthy blood-sugar control is key to weight management post-menopause. Insulin resistance makes your body start relying more on glucose because high insulin supresses fat burning (it affects those mTOR and AMPK pathways), which is why it can be so hard to lose weight. Insulin resistance can then mean more energy crashes, instances of 'hanger', feeling tired even after eating and that stubborn weight around the middle. But there is much we can do to work with these metabolic changes at midlife.

changes in fat deposition

During the menopause transition, the reduction in oestrogen can cause more visceral weight gain – around the middle – which is more metabolically dysregulated. Visceral fat is very different to the subcutaneous fat found on our lower body (hips and thighs), which is more metabolically protective. Visceral fat can increase by up to 50 per cent during the perimenopause transition and can start to produce inflammatory markers. Inflammation, as we know, is a key player in chronic disease. It can worsen insulin resistance, oxidize LDL cholesterol (which makes it more likely to stick to artery walls) and trigger the immune system. Reduced oestrogen levels can reduce our ability to burn fats for fuel, through a process called beta-oxidation. High insulin can prevent fat burning; fat is directed instead towards cholesterol synthesis and fat deposition. This means that triglycerides in the blood increase, including LDL cholesterol. Consisting of what are known as 'small, dense LDL particles', tiny bits of these particles can come loose and become lodged within blood vessel walls. This is why there is such a connection between our metabolic health and our cardiovascular risk. More on cholesterol in the next chapter.

longevity larder

SEEDS

All seeds are brilliant sources of plant-based protein, fibre, vitamin E, minerals and plant-based beneficial fats, including omega 6 (especially sunflower, pumpkin and hemp seeds) and omega-3 (the greatest source being linseed/flaxseed). Sesame seeds are one of the oldest oilseed crops and are a good source of minerals such as zinc, as well as sesamin, a lignan polyphenol. Chia seeds were used as early as 3,500 BCE in Central and South America; the name *chia* is the Mayan word for 'strength'. Fresh linseed/flaxseed oil is a great source of omega-3, which in its plant form is called alpha-linolenic acid and has been shown in many studies to help reduce LDL cholesterol and slow cardiovascular progression.[32] Alpha-linolenic acid is converted to EPA and DHA, which have anti-inflammatory effects on the body. Ground linseed is very much part of my post-menopausal toolkit because it not only provides plenty of soluble fibre, which massages your gut on the way down and helps supports cholesterol levels, it's also a wonderful source of phytoestrogens in the form of lignans. Pop 2 tablespoons on your high-protein granola or porridge, or into your overnight oats.

how to lose weight sustainably post-menopause

First things first, we don't want to fall into the diet trap...especially when we are post-menopause! Our focus is on those metabolic pathways and helping to support fat burn at the same time as muscle growth. We want to change up our diet to include more foods that are full of nutrients, protein and beneficial fats and fibre in order to support our bones, our heart and our brain too. A highly restrictive, low fat (low joy!) diet is not helpful. Restricting food can reduce our metabolic rate and deplete our energy, which isn't going to make us want to move more. I often want my clients to eat more – but more helpful foods. This is when dieting is just not supportive for us.

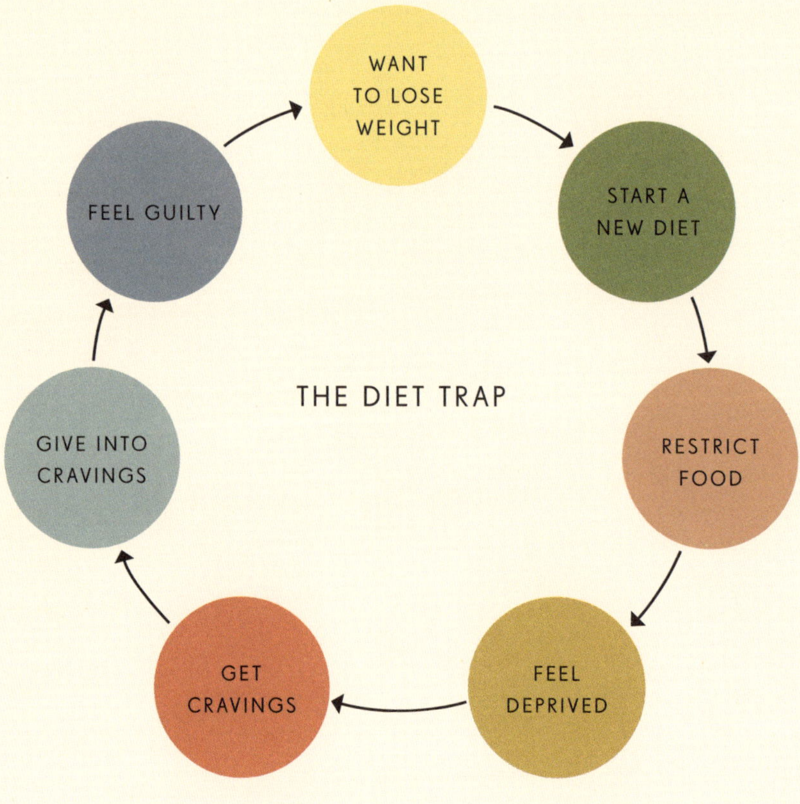

When we fall into the diet trap, we often feel like we are battling our body and its stubborn weight gain. Now is the time to start giving our body some grace, and celebrating all that it has gone through to get to this point – as well as the fact that it now carries us post-menopause, which as we know, is a privilege many don't get. There is a lot of language and guilt related to food that we have often carried around with us for many years – even coming from childhood, especially if we had a mother who was constantly dieting or commenting on our size. The kind of language we should ditch includes 'diet', 'treat', 'being naughty', 'cheat day', referencing how many Slimming World Syns are in a food or drink, 'good and bad food', and getting rid of that moral superiority we think comes with being thin. Dieting takes up too much time: weighing food or counting calories or Syns, worrying about social events and what we are going to eat – or maybe not eating all day because of an event – and seeing food and movement as transactional. Dieting can often make our food choices too complex, too restrictive and, in some cases, too costly. I want food always to be seen as celebration. Now it is time to change the narrative and give yourself permission to enjoy food!

I like to reframe good or bad food as helpful versus less helpful. I eat both, but for the main part, the food I eat is helpful. Not because I have a halo permanently over my head, but because I crave nutritious food most of the time, which this section of the book will help you achieve too. My focus for sustainable weight loss is always on being healthy and happy without dieting, or guilt! Understanding what is going on at menopause, why we can put this weight on around the middle and why it is so hard to get rid of, is key to giving ourselves some grace. The body views excess weight as a survival mechanism, in case there are times of famine ahead. Human biology hasn't really changed much for millennia, but we are dealing with a food supply very different to the one we were biochemically programmed for! Sustainable change is what we are after, so that we minimize the loss of lean muscle mass and focus on fat loss, not weight loss. Losing around one to two pounds per week reduces the risk of losing muscle mass, so this is what we should be aiming for.

Weight-bearing exercise can also help to protect our lean muscle mass post-menopause, to keep us strong and reduce the risk of becoming frail later in life. This is a crucial part of the midlife weight-loss toolkit – essential to do alongside the dietary changes outlined here. Ideally two to three times a week. It's amazing how quickly you can build up your weights. Muscles are more metabolically active, too – muscle tissue burns more calories than fat. However, as I tell my clients, I prefer to see weight loss as a nice side benefit of weight training, with the main aim being increased energy and strength, in addition to improvements in sleep, digestion and mood. This approach helps us to value what we are gaining rather than thinking about how much weight we are losing – a much more positive way to see things. It also means that we build more sustainable habits in place of yo-yo dieting or feeling guilty about what we are eating. The focus should always be about what you can add in to reduce the cravings for less helpful food.

Protein is our fat-loss power food. It is essential for many things related to weight loss. Protein is more satiating than other macronutrients, so it helps to anchor our hunger, regulate our appetite, support insulin sensitivity and crowd out sugar cravings. It helps us to fast for longer, which means more fat burn on the AMPK pathway – supporting that metabolic flexibility. Protein is made up of amino acids, which are the 'building blocks' of the body, supporting organs, skin and muscles. Protein is therefore essential for preserving our lean muscle mass as we lose weight. Muscles act like a sponge for excess glucose, too, so greater muscle mass is hugely important to combat insulin resistance. Higher protein is also a good source of collagen, which helps support our musculoskeletal system post-menopause. Aim for a palm-sized portion of a high-protein food with every meal: lean meat, poultry, eggs, tofu, tempeh, dairy products, oily fish, nuts and seeds, beans, lentils, quinoa and yogurt.

High-fibre foods also support satiety – fibre is a natural GLP-1 inducer! High-fibre foods can slow down digestion and increase the stretch receptors in the stomach that signal that we are full. This leads to fewer cravings and less hunger. Soluble fibre from oats, legumes and ground linseed/flaxseed, for example, not only delays gastric emptying but also helps reduce cholesterol levels. Fibre feeds the beneficial bacteria in the gut. Fermentation of fibre produces short-chain fatty acids like butyrate, which has been shown to improve insulin sensitivity and regulate leptin and ghrelin via the gut–brain axis. A high-fibre diet is linked to reduced visceral fat and better blood-sugar regulation.

Try to be more carb-conscious, too, make sure carbohydrate sources like rice or gluten-free pasta only fill around a quarter of your plate. Also reduce refined carb sources like biscuits, bread, bagels, breakfast cereals, cakes and pastries. For example, a handful of dry white rice constitutes a

longevity larder

CHICKPEAS (PULSES)

Chickpeas are thought to have been cultivated in what is now Turkey and Syria as long ago as 7500 BCE, eventually spreading to many other locations in the Middle East, North Africa and Asia. They're also known as garbanzo beans, Bengal gram, Egyptian peas, ceci beans and Kabuli chana. Aside from beige they can be black, green, red or brown. Chickpeas are a great source of fibre, which is often low in our diets. They are also a rich source of a particular carbohydrate (an oligosaccharide) called raffinose. Raffinose is known as a prebiotic – it helps to create the right environment in our guts for beneficial bacteria to grow. Aside from providing plant-based protein and iron, chickpeas are also a great source of non-dairy calcium and are rich in magnesium and B6, essential for energy, hormone balance and sleep.

single portion. Opt for brown rice or wild rice over white, too, whenever you can. Make the meal about the protein and the vegetables, rather than the pasta, rice or potatoes. Making more dishes using tofu and tempeh, nuts, seeds, yogurt and pulses is a great plant-based way to up our protein content. Replacing pasta with quinoa, or even edamame pasta, which is high in phytoestrogens, is another useful way of getting more protein onto our plates. Focus more on complex carbs, too, including brown rice, lentils and other pulses, squash and sweet potato, and even potato salad. Cooked and cooled potatoes give us something called resistant starch, which is a prebiotic and helps support our gut bacteria.

Extra virgin olive oil polyphenols (especially oleuropein) have been shown to activate the AMPK fat-burning pathway. This improves the ability of the cells in our body and brain to use fat as energy. It enhances mitochondrial efficiency (our cells' energy factories) and reduces the inflammation that goes hand in hand with metabolic imbalances.

longevity larder

CINNAMON (SPICES)

Cinnamon was once as valuable as gold. It's a spice obtained from the inner bark of the *Cinnamomum* tree. Cinnamon has been used for thousands of years to help calm digestive problems, and recent research indicates that cinnamon may also help the body to balance its energy reserves between meals by helping lowering blood sugar. There are many compounds in cinnamon, including polyphenols, and cinnamaldehyde, cinnamic acid and cinnamate. One of the polyphenols is type-A procyanidin oligomer, responsible for cinnamon's antioxidant and insulin-like benefits for balancing blood sugar. Both cinnamaldehyde and cinnamic acid have antifungal and antimicrobial properties, and cinnamic acid also has anti-inflammatory benefits. Cinnamic acid and cinnamate contribute to the spice's flavour. Opt for Ceylon cinnamon from Sri Lanka rather than cassia cinnamon, which is grown in China, Vietnam and elsewhere; because Ceylon cinnamon has less coumarin in it, which can be toxic at high dosages.

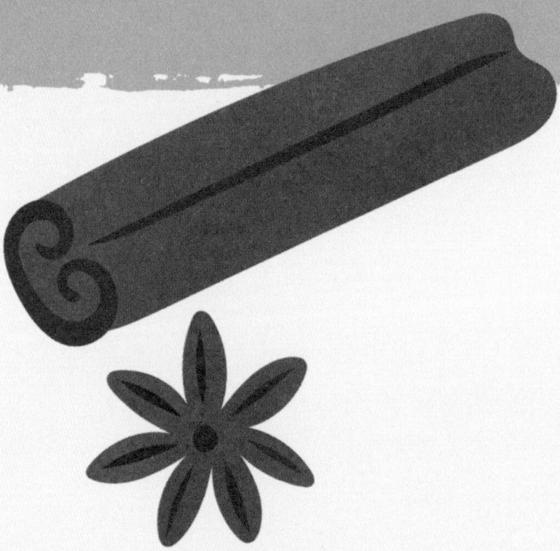

fasting and meal timing

Fasting has been shown to help reduce metabolic issues and increase longevity. In a fasted state, insulin drops, fat cells release stored fatty acids, and the liver turns these fats into fuel. Food noise quietens because the body is no longer panicking about its next carbohydrate fix – it's happily burning its own stored fuel. Ideally, a fasting window of around 14 hours overnight is most beneficial, with four-hour fasts between meals. Mini-fasts between meals helps to reduce insulin release. The more insulin release there is, the more we increase fat storage, and the higher the risk of developing insulin resistance. Combine fasted periods with a walk or some other light aerobic exercise to further encourage fat mobilization. This should all help to control appetite and support healthy metabolic function.

Breakfast like a queen! So many of us who want to lose weight – well, fat – don't eat breakfast and often backload most of our calories to the second half of the day, which is counterproductive for weight loss. If you are following the 16:8 fasting regime, then enjoy breakfast at 9:30am and an early dinner at 5:30pm and go to bed a bit hungry. People living in the Blue Zones all eat like this. We also used to eat like this – the full English breakfast! Where we would fuel ourselves to support a busy day, often involving manual labour. All this has changed now – we grab a coffee first thing, which stops us from feeling hungry (and we often don't wake up hungry because we've eaten our evening meal so late), so we don't want to eat until mid-morning, if not later. Then we have a massive crash in the afternoon because we haven't fuelled ourselves well enough at the start of the day, and then we can't stop eating. There is a lot of research on how eating a fuller breakfast improves satiety through the rest of the day. Aim to have 20 to 25 grams of protein for breakfast. Examples include: two large eggs, 1 tbsp pumpkin seeds, half a small avocado (50g) and one slice of seeded sourdough (26g total protein), or mix 150g 0%-fat Greek yoghurt with 120ml unsweetened soya milk, 1 tbsp chia seeds, 1 tbsp ground linseed/flaxseed, cinnamon, a handful blueberries, 1 tbsp almond butter and 1 tbsp mixed seeds (30g protein).

the concept of *hara hachi bu* and other mindfulness techniques

Hara hachi bu is a 2,500-year-old Confucian teaching followed by Okinawans – meaning eating until you are 80 per cent full. Other cultures around the world also have similar phrases. We often forget about the wisdom of this! A lot of the time we don't even let ourselves get hungry anymore. Try to bring a bit more mindfulness to your eating routine. Eat slower – so many of us inhale our food! Slowing down reduces the risk of overeating. A three-day food and drink diary can be a really useful exercise – not to judge yourself but just to bring some focus to what you have been eating. So many of us have eating routines that are very passive – we are not even aware we are eating! Smaller plates are also something to think about – sometimes the dishes we use are huge. Portions-wise, look to have a palm-sized serving each of protein and veg, a fist-sized serving of carbohydrates and a thumb-sized serving of healthy fats – your nuts and seeds and olive oil. Try not to eat in front of a screen or on the go. Think about what you are going to eat for your evening meal at the start of the day so that you can pick up any missing ingredients during the day and take anything needed out of the freezer to defrost. I'm not one for batch cooking but I often eat leftovers from my evening meal the next day for lunch.

kuchisabishii – how to overcome emotional eating

Do you only ever eat because you are hungry, or do you sometimes eat because you feel bored or stressed or sad, or because you've had a bad (or even a good) day – or for several of these reasons combined? There is a great Japanese expression, *kuchisabishii*, meaning 'lonely mouth', that I think sums up emotional eating brilliantly – we eat because our mouths are lonely! And of course, emotional eating isn't satisfied by food either. We are reaching for food when what we really need is comfort or an escape from those negative emotions. My first bit of advice is to be aware of it when it happens, with no self-judgement, and to know what your cues are: is it a certain time of day? After work? Or when commuting? Or do you stress eat? Once you identify the trigger, you can change up the reward – if it tends to happen in the evening, then take a magnesium salt bath to help calm your nervous system rather than reaching for food, then put your pyjamas on and brush your teeth. Or post-bath, go enjoy some sofa time and have a herbal tea. If it's on the commute, take a flask of hot water and lemon to drink on the train – buying coffee at the station might have strong associations with eating pastries or other less helpful foods. Whereas you could have a lovely Blackberry, Acai and Cacao Chia Pot (see recipe on p.149) in your bag to enjoy at work with your coffee.

the problem with alcohol

The liver prioritizes the removal of alcohol over everything else! I am not the alcohol police, but I thought it was important to discuss a little about its effects on us metabolically. Alcohol disrupts our sleep massively – if we experience low blood sugar in the night, this can wake us up, due to the release of stress hormones to balance blood glucose. Lack of sleep then affects our insulin resistance the next day. We also have to deal with a hangover, which means we're more likely to crave carbs and caffeine. We know that alcohol fuels anxiety, too – hence the term 'hangxeity'. Zinc is often known as the anti-anxiety mineral because it helps support the production of the brain's primary calming neurochemical, GABA. Good levels of zinc not only support GABA production, they also inhibit the opposing more excitory neurochemical glutamate. When we drink alcohol, GABA increases and glutamate decreases in the short term, which is why alcohol can make us feel relaxed. However, glutamate is then released after we stop drinking, as the brain compensates for lower levels, which can then make us feel jangly and anxious. Having a magnesium salt bath is great for properly calming the nervous system in the same way alcohol *seems* to do (because it is actually a stimulant). Unfortunately, we live in a culture where alcohol is very much front and centre but thankfully now there are far more of us who are 'sober curious', and there are lots of lovely non-alcoholic drinks out there that will give you that feeling of having something alcoholic but without the hangover.

nutritional shifts:

- Breakfast like a queen! And make it high in protein sources.
- Eat more protein with every meal to support lean muscle growth: lean meat, fish, eggs, dairy, soy, nuts, seeds and pulses.
- Increase fibre-rich foods – aim for 30+ different plants a week. There are lots of plant-based recipes for you to try in the recipe section.
- Be carb conscious – focus on complex carbohydrates.
- Don't avoid all fats – up your beneficial monounsaturated fats (extra virgin olive oil), and omega-3 and 6 fatty acids such as oily fish, nuts and seeds, linseed/flaxseed; avocados, and Greek yogurt or probiotic yogurt (sweeten it yourself).
- Use extra virgin olive oil in your cooking – fats are essential for the absorption of the fat-soluble vitamins A, D, E and K.
- Avoid ultra-processed foods and anything containing artificial sweeteners, which can artificially create more hunger cues after eating them.
- Remember the AMPK pathway supporters: chilli, the quercetin flavonoid (found in onions, leeks, apples and grapes) and green tea.
- Include healthy fats (olive oil, nuts, avocados) to promote satiety.
- Include natural GLP-1 inhibitors in the form of high-fibre foods: oats, barley, pulses, brassicas, carrots and sweet potatoes, and high protein foods such as chicken, turkey, fish, eggs, tofu and pulses.
- Add cinnamon to support insulin sensitivity.
- Chromium is a micromineral known to do the same.
- Enjoy a little of what you fancy!

lifestyle shifts:

- Eat at similar times of the day and aim for three meals a day.
- Eat earlier in the evening.
- Practise mindful eating – chew your food well and don't eat in front of a screen.
- No eating on the go, which makes us less mindful.
- No snacking.
- Think about what you are going to cook for dinner first thing so you can make sure you get ingredients defrosted and pick up what you are missing during the day.
- Aim to fast for 14 hours overnight – water and herbal teas are fine to have.
- Start (or increase) weight training – around three times a week, if you can.
- Consistency over perfection always!

supplements to consider:

(Not to be taken all together, and if you are on any medication, do speak to your healthcare practitioner before starting any new supplements)

There are no magic weight-loss supplements, but I would recommend a good all-round multi to supply you with plenty of vitamins, minerals and antioxidants to help support your metabolism.

- BioCare, Menopause Multinutrient
- Together Health, Menopause Multivitamin
- Wild Nutrition, Weight Management Support

queen of hearts

HOW TO SUPPORT OUR CARDIOVASCULAR HEALTH

So, on to matters of the heart. What a workhorse the heart is, pumping around 7,000 litres of blood every day! Our heart health is also affected by the stressors of midlife: dealing with teens, elderly parents, grief, divorce, sexism, racism, lack of time, work and financial stressors, and then menopause on top of this. The risk of a heart attack increases significantly post-menopause becoming the same as a man's – in fact more women die of cardiovascular disease (CVD) than from all forms of cancer combined, which is pretty shocking. Heart attacks in women are 50 per cent more likely to be misdiagnosed than in men – our symptoms are often different, so can be missed.[33] These can include: shortness of breath, nausea, vomiting and cold sweats, overwhelming weakness or fatigue, anxiety, lethargy, loss of appetite, and pain in the jaw, back or neck. Our blood pressure and cholesterol levels can increase post-menopause too. However, it is estimated that a whopping 80 to 90 per cent of our CVD risk is preventable through diet and lifestyle shifts,[34] which is HUGE! It's so empowering to know that we can do something about it. We can adapt!

Let's firstly look at why our cardiovascular health (our heart, blood and blood vessels) can change during menopause. Menopause is now classified as an inflammatory transitional event in our lives,[35] while inflammation is one of the key drivers of CVD.[36] Oestrogen exerts an anti-inflammatory effect on the body (although it has pro-inflammatory roles too, so it's not entirely straightforward). When oestrogen levels are high, it helps to dilate our blood vessels, and when they dip, it constricts them. This is why heart palpitations are a common symptom during perimenopause and why women have a higher risk of developing high blood pressure and CVD post-menopause.[37] Our cholesterol levels may also increase. One factor might be lower oestrogen, which helps to support the removal of low-density lipoprotein (LDL) cholesterol. Oestrogen helps increase LDL receptor expression on the surface of the liver, which removes LDL from the blood for processing. LDL is often known as 'bad' cholesterol. It transports cholesterol to where it's needed around the body, but too much can lead to a build-up in blood-vessel walls, increasing the risk of heart attacks and strokes. Other considerations also impact our LDL cholesterol levels and overall cardiovascular health, and many of these are related to our metabolic health. How your body responds to insulin is a key factor in metabolic health. Insulin resistance can increase blood-sugar levels, inflammation and oxidative stress and blood lipids. It can also lead to higher LDL cholesterol and lower HDL cholesterol ('good' cholesterol, which travels around the bloodstream picking up excess cholesterol and taking it to the liver for recycling or removal), as well as changes in LDL (a process called glycation, which makes LDL more susceptible to oxidation and can damage blood vessels). This is why there is such a connection between our cardiovascular and metabolic health – the cardiometabolic connection.

Cholesterol is not the bad guy! It's part of every cell membrane in the body and is an essential precursor for vitamin D synthesis and for all our steroid hormones, for bile acids to help break down fats, and it makes up part of the brain fat too (which is why offal/brains are so high in cholesterol, not something that I will be recommending…). Most of our cholesterol (around 80 per cent) is made in the liver. Our liver is therefore our primary source of cholesterol, not our diet. High LDL but low Apolipoprotein B (ApoB) particles is now regarded as a better predicator of cardiovascular risk. A low ApoB level with high LDL can indicate that the cholesterol is packed into fewer, larger particles (lower risk) rather than many small particles (higher risk).[38] Cholesterol isn't bad, but its oxidation is, and we can do something about this. It's important to note, though, that we can't reduce the risk of CVD to just high cholesterol or lower oestrogen levels. There are lots of other factors involved, including oxidative stress, obesity, high blood pressure, poor circulation, high levels of calcium (which can cause calcification of arteries – usually from high-calcium supplements without cofactors), low nutrient intake, alcohol and smoking. Much can be done to support our cardiovascular health in this post-menopause window, adapting to the changes in oestrogen and metabolism by making small changes to our lifestyle and diet.

anti-inflammatory foods

CVD is classified as being inflammatory in nature and, as we know, menopause is now considered an inflammatory event in a woman's life. Chronic inflammation plays a key role in atherosclerosis – the build-up of fatty material or plaque inside the blood vessels, which can lead to heart attacks and strokes. This is why foods that exert an anti-inflammatory effect on the body are incredibly important for our cardiovascular health post-menopause. If you reduce inflammation, you can improve blood-vessel flexibility. Omega-3 fatty acids are one of the key nutrients exerting an anti-inflammatory effect – they've been shown to help keep LDL

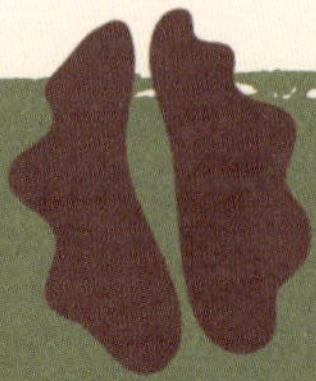

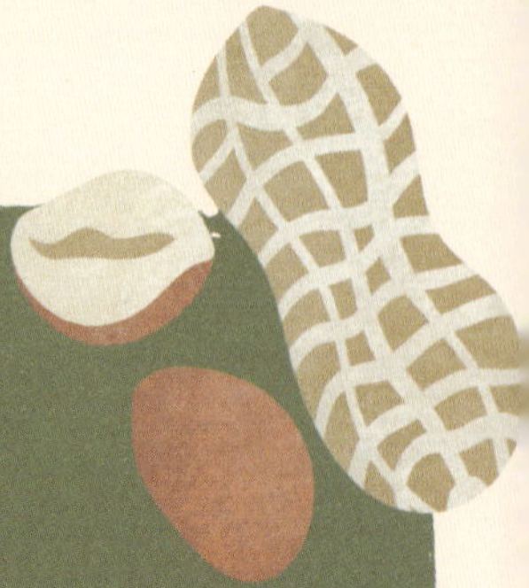

longevity larder

NUTS

Nuts are an anti-inflammatory powerhouse! A study has shown that regularly eating nuts is associated with a lower risk of heart disease.[40] A trial held in Spain from 2003 to 2011 (PREDIMED) to assess the benefits of the Mediterranean diet found that older adults at higher risk of CVD who followed the diet enriched with nuts had a 30 per cent CVD risk reduction after just four years compared to those on a standard low-fat diet.[41] Walnuts are a great source of flavonoids – especially the wispy paper-like parts that are revealed when you crack open a whole nut – while almonds provide vitamin E, a potent antioxidant vitamin. Brazil nuts are a great source of selenium, an essential mineral for creating the powerful antioxidant glutathione peroxidase, and for the optimal function of superoxide dismutase, another antioxidant produced by the body. Both are hugely important for preventing the oxidation of LDL cholesterol.[42]

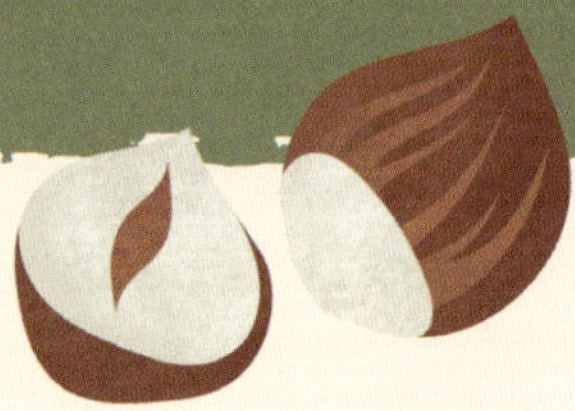

in check, and to keep blood vessels and cell membranes healthy and flexible.[39] Sources of omega-3 include oily fish, such as salmon, sardines and mackerel. Nuts, seeds and linseed/flaxseed oil are also great plant-based sources.

Turmeric and ginger are part of the polyphenol family – potent anti-inflammatories known to benefit our cardiovascular health. Ginger is known to reduce arterial plaque, preventing platelet aggregation, which leads to blood clots.[43] Turmeric has been shown to reduce oxidative stress and improve vasodilation.[44] Polyphenols, like anthocyanins, protect against the inflammation that contributes to heart disease, due to their antioxidant capabilities. They are found in berries, cherries and beetroot,[45] and work with our gut microbes to reduce inflammation,

longevity larder

GINGER

Used in Ayurvedic and Traditional Chinese Medicine for over 5,000 years, ginger helps to combat nausea, reduce inflammation, support the 'fire' of the digestive system (stomach acid) and aid the joints due to its now well-researched anti-inflammatory action. The active constituents of ginger include gingerols and shogaols. These phytonutrients are used by the roots to fend off invaders – and they do the same for us. *Shringavera*, the name for ginger in Sanskrit, means 'horn' – a great description of its shape!

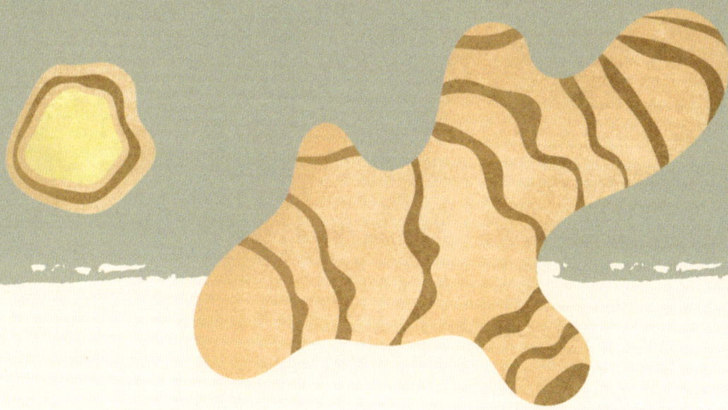

improve blood-vessel flexibility, and protect brain and muscle cells. Several randomized controlled trials have suggested that regular consumption of blueberries may protect against cognitive decline and help lower blood pressure in post-menopausal women with above-normal blood pressure.[46]

Fibre supports a healthy gut microbiome – also connected to our heart health. Research suggests that gut health can be an important driver of CVD because gut dysbiosis can be such a site of inflammation.[47] The gut microbiome acts like a control centre for our metabolism and immune system. Bacteria in the gut metabolize certain nutrients, such as choline, betaine and L-carnitine, into trimethylamine-N-oxide (TMAO). High levels of TMAO have been associated with an increased risk of CVD.[48]

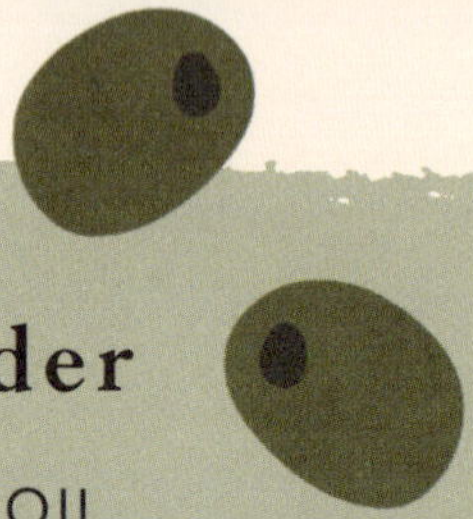

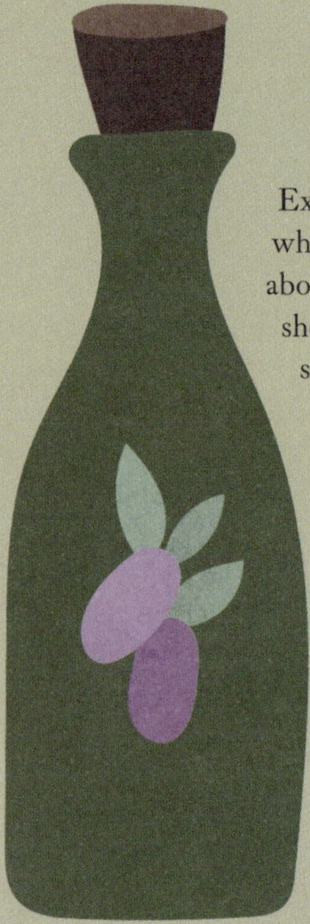

longevity larder

EXTRA VIRGIN OLIVE OIL

Extra virgin olive oil (EVOO) contains hydroxytyrosol, which is one of the most powerful antioxidants we know about. High-quality, extra virgin olive oil should taste fresh, should be green-ish in colour and slightly bitter, all of which signal high hydroxytyrosol content. EVOO also contains a compound called oleocanthal, which accounts for the peppery taste – the fresher the olive oil the more likely you are to get this stronger taste. Oleocanthal exerts anti-inflammatory effects similar to ibuprofen (it downregulates COX-1 and COX-2 pro-inflammatory pathways), which is why EVOO is so central to the anti-inflammatory effects of the Mediterranean diet. The polyphenol content acts as a defence against LDL cholesterol oxidation too. Always buy it in a dark glass bottle – too much light and it will oxidize. It is a monounsaturated fat, so for most cooking heats it's fine to use and doesn't oxidize.

The Mediterranean diet was first researched back in the 1950s due to low instances of cardiovascular disease in the region. So, what makes it so cardioprotective? One of the most important heart-healthy elements of the diet is the extra virgin olive oil.

Tomatoes are rich in lycopene, another polyphenol, and these are another important component of the Mediterranean diet. Low blood levels of lycopene have been linked to an increased risk of heart attack and stroke.[49] Lycopene can help stabilize cholesterol by reducing the negative effects of lipid oxidation – done by helping to neutralize the impact of excess free-radical production. Garlic, too, has long been studied for its blood-pressure and cholesterol-lowering effects.[50]

longevity larder

GARLIC
(BRIGHTLY COLOURED VEGETABLES, INCLUDING WHITE!)

Related to onions, leeks and chives, garlic was called the 'great panacea' by the Greek physician Galen, as well as 'Russian penicillin', due to its use in Russia as an antimicrobial during World War 2. Thought to have originated in Siberia, it was also used as a remedy in ancient China. Over 100 different compounds have been identified in garlic, including S-allyl cysteine, which is well absorbed and may well account for some of the health benefits attributed to garlic. Hippocrates mentioned garlic as a remedy against intestinal parasites, and even today it's used to combat parasites and as an antifungal. Ancient wisdom indeed! Allicin and ajoene are thought to be responsible for garlic's antifungal activity. Chopping fresh garlic activates allicin. Wait five minutes after chopping before adding to acidic foods (such as tomatoes and lemon juice) as acid deactivates the enzymatic process. Cooking also deactivates allicin, so it is best enjoyed raw – pesto and salsa verde are great options, and there are lots of recipes in this book to enjoy it this way.

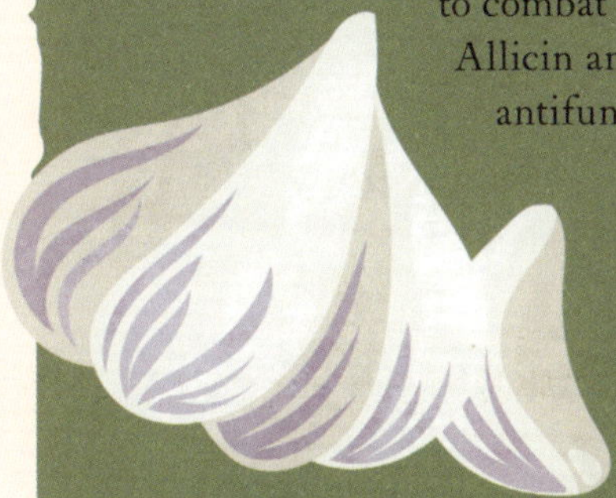

HERBS FOR HEART HARMONY: SUPPORTING CIRCULATION AND VITALITY FOR LIFE

Melinda McDougall
Medical Herbalist, MSc, MNIMH

As we move through menopause and beyond, protecting our hearts and cardiovascular system becomes a priority. Botanical medicines complement conventional approaches and provide unique preventative health benefits. Many herbs contain complex phytochemicals that have vasodilatory, antioxidant, anti-inflammatory and cardiotonic actions. Unlike isolated pharmaceutical compounds that may have a singular mode of action, medicinal plants work synergistically with the body, gently reinforcing cardiovascular function and protecting vascular integrity.

Some of the herbal medicines I use in my women's health clinic to help support cardiovascular health are listed below. Most of them have been used by herbalists, apothecaries and physicians for hundreds of years – and science is increasingly catching up with research studies confirming their value. Be mindful of interactions with prescription medication and always consult a medical herbalist for individual advice.

Hawthorn (*Crataegus* spp.) is arguably the most important cardiovascular herb in European herbal medicine. The berries, leaves and flowers contain flavonoids and oligomeric proanthocyanidins, which enhance myocardial oxygen utilization, increase coronary blood flow, and improve the strength of cardiac contractility. Hawthorn has a gentle tonic effect on the cardiac muscle, improving function in cases of mild hypertension, early congestive heart failure and age-related decline in cardiac efficiency. Its long safety record and mild cumulative action make it particularly valuable in preventative care for our ageing physiology. And it's freely and abundantly available in our hedgerows, giving us swathes of beautiful creamy flowers across the countryside each spring, and radiant red berries in autumn.

Where hawthorn strengthens, **yarrow (*Achillea millefolium*)** regulates and refines. Traditionally known as an external wound herb, yarrow also works internally to support the fine architecture of the circulatory system. Rich in volatile oils, sesquiterpene lactones and flavonoids, yarrow improves peripheral circulation and optimizes vascular tone. It helps moderate mild hypertension through its vasodilatory actions and supports blood-vessel integrity by reducing capillary fragility. For those with compromised microcirculation – often experienced as cold extremities, varicose veins or slow wound healing – yarrow can be an important supportive herb.

Rhodiola (*Rhodiola rosea*), best known as an adaptogen for stamina and stress resilience, shows promising cardioprotective qualities. By supporting healthier stress responses and calming over-active sympathetic nervous system drive, Rhodiola helps ease the burden that chronic tension places on the heart and blood vessels. Its active constituents appear to shield heart tissue from oxidative stress and maintain the integrity of the vascular lining, helping to protect against the gradual wear-and-tear that contributes to vascular ageing. Studies suggest that Rhodiola may help the heart recover from periods of low oxygen supply, stabilize blood-pressure responses and preserve healthy circulation. Where cardiovascular risks are intertwined with stress, fatigue and emotional strain (hello menopause), Rhodiola serves as a restorative ally, helping nurture long-term heart resilience and vitality.

Ginger (*Zingiber officinale*) is warming, enlivening and deeply nourishing. Its anti-inflammatory and antiplatelet properties can help reduce cardiovascular risk, while also improving peripheral circulation. Known primarily as a digestive stimulant, this resilient root contains gingerols and shogaols that help reduce blood clotting, improve blood flow and encourage healthy vascular responsiveness. As a culinary and medicinal herb, it's one we can all integrate into our daily lives by adding it to recipes, or simply grating fresh ginger into a cup of hot water – perfect on a winter's morning.

Ginkgo (*Ginkgo biloba*), one of our oldest living tree species, is renowned for its effects on cerebral microcirculation, helping maintain clarity, memory and cognitive vitality – but it is also beneficial for the entire vascular system. Ginkgo enhances endothelial function, improves blood flow and supports microvascular integrity. Its antioxidant properties help reduce damage to vessels – a core factor in atherosclerosis and age-related arterial stiffening. It inhibits platelet aggregation – simply meaning it stops the blood from clotting – which is key to preventing strokes. I also find it beneficial for tinnitus. It's an all-round winner for the ageing brain and circulatory system. Seek advice if already taking anticoagulant medication.

For a calming cardiotonic herb, look no further than **motherwort (*Leonurus cardiaca*)**. This is my 'go to' herb for menopausal heart palpitations (when all other causes have been ruled out). For those whose cardiovascular symptoms are intertwined with stress, grief or worry, motherwort reminds the heart to slow down, breathe and find its rhythm again. Iridoid glycosides and alkaloids impart gentle anti-arrhythmic effects, steadying an over-rapid pulse and reducing racing heartbeats. With a Latin name featuring the word *cardiaca*, this is grounding, soothing and strengthening medicine for the heart.

Where circulation feels slow and stagnant, **prickly ash (*Zanthoxylum americanum*)** serves as a sparky stimulant. The bark of this native North American tree has been used for centuries to improve circulation to the capillary networks found in our extremities. Particularly useful for those with cold hands and feet, varicose veins or poor circulation resulting in skin ulcers or wounds, it helps oxygenate tissues and improve vascular tone. It has similar properties to the **horse chestnut (*Aesculus hippocastanum*)** tree – the seeds of which make a powerful tonic for the vascular system that can be used internally (in tincture or supplement form) or externally, as a cream or lotion. Think of this next time you are throwing a conker!

Rosemary (*Rosmarinus officinalis*) stimulates cerebral circulation, supports antioxidant defence of the arterial lining and encourages healthy lipid metabolism – an important factor in maintaining arterial health across the ageing process and through menopause. Traditionally associated with memory and vitality, it clears the mind and lifts our spirits. Simply crush its leaves and breathe in those volatile oils to understand its potent effect on mental function.

Finally, the honey-scented **Limeflower (*Tilia* spp.)** offers gentle sedative, vasodilatory, and antispasmodic actions that aid the cardiovascular system indirectly by helping to modulate stress responses and tension-induced blood-pressure elevation. Known as the linden tree across Europe, its sticky, sweet flowers are famed for their relaxing properties and as an after-dinner tea. As chronic stress and sympathetic dominance are well-documented contributors to cardiovascular disease, limeflower's ability to soothe the nervous system and support vascular relaxation makes it an excellent herb for preventative cardiovascular care.

By harnessing traditional wisdom enhanced by emerging research, we can support our ageing hearts and embrace not only longer life, but healthier and more vibrant living.

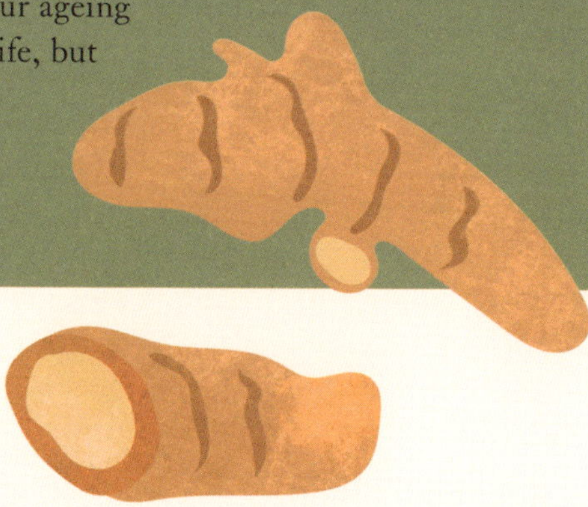

springtime hawthorn blossom cordial

100g/3 ½oz golden caster sugar
500ml/17fl oz filtered water
100g/3 ½oz hawthorn flowers
1 lemon

When the hawthorn blooms in springtime, pick the blossoms early in the morning when they are fresh – watch out for the thorns. Wash and remove any insects. Mix the sugar and water in a saucepan and simmer until all the sugar is dissolved. Remove from the heat and add the flowers – crush them a little to release more of their flavour. Slice the lemon and add to the mixture. Cover and leave to infuse for up to 4 hours. Remove the lemon slices and strain through muslin into a clean jug and pour into sterilized jars or bottles. Store in the fridge. Add a dash to tonic or soda and ice for a refreshing spring tonic that strengthens the heart. In summer, you can re-create this recipe using limeflowers instead.

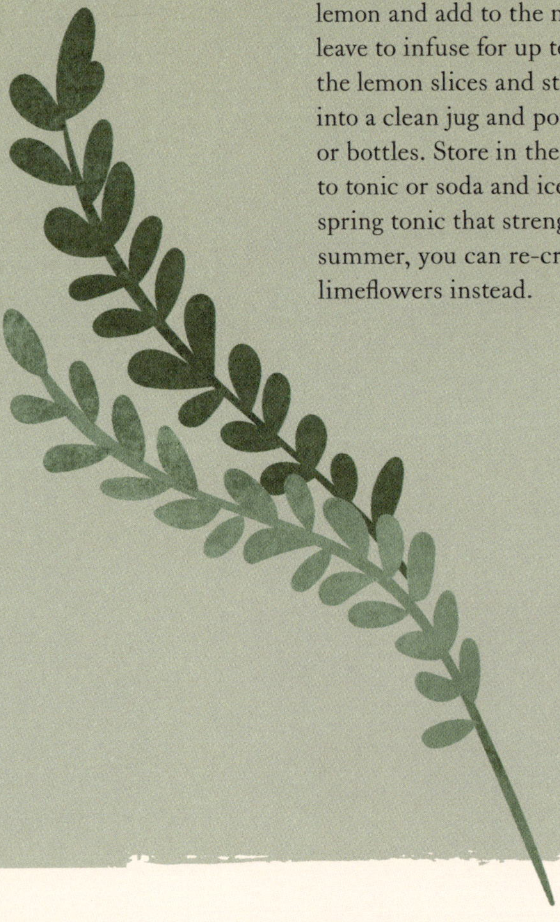

other key nutrients

A 2025 review highlighted the many ways that phytoestrogens may exert their cardioprotective effect,[51] and a recent observational study in Asia showed that dietary intake of soy isoflavones had a significant inverse association with coronary heart disease.[52] This family of plants are known to support vasodilation and also have beneficial effects on cholesterol due to their plant sterol content, which can block cholesterol absorption in the gut. Isoflavones found in soy and lignans found in plants such as linseed, are polyphenols with an antioxidant effect.

Calcium and magnesium are minerals that are hugely important for balancing the rhythm of the heart, and abnormally low or high levels of either of them can cause arrhythmia, while low magnesium has been shown to cause heart palpitations.[53] Although a Western diet tends to provide adequate amounts of calcium, low vitamin D can reduce absorption, leading to low calcium levels. Potassium is another vital mineral, but a Western diet can be low in this (something that also corresponds with high sodium levels; see p.71). The best sources of potassium are plants, especially vegetables. This is why green leafy vegetables are so important for our cardiovascular health – they provide us with calcium, magnesium, potassium, folate and vitamin C, which are all really important heart-health nutrients. Higher vitamin C status is associated with lower risks of hypertension, coronary heart disease and stroke.[54] Vitamin C is important for helping with vasodilation; it is an important antioxidant too.

Between 1993 and 1998, a study of 29,689 Italian women showed a high intake of leafy green vegetables (and olive oil) was linked to a significantly lower risk of coronary heart disease.[55] Green leafy vegetables are high in vitamin B9 (folate), which is required to break down an amino acid called homocysteine. Homocysteine levels that are too high can increase the risk of heart attack and stroke. B9, B12 and B6 break homocysteine down into other amino acids: methionine (as part of the methionine cycle, part of methylation ; pp.18–19) and cysteine, made from methionine. Cysteine has anti-inflammatory effects and methionine is an antioxidant. This is why these B vitamins are so crucial to not only our cardiovascular health but to our longevity too. Eat your greens!

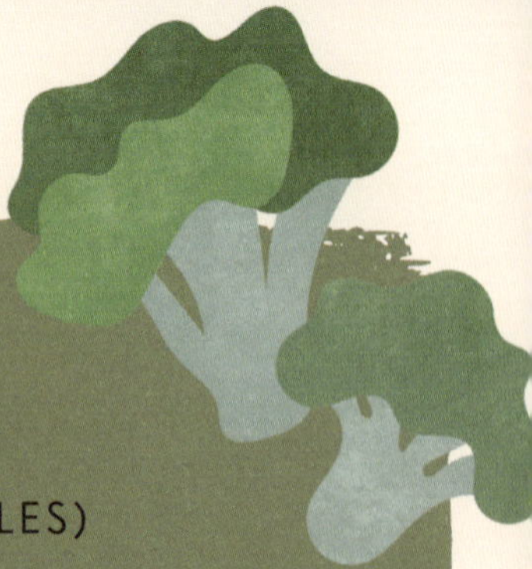

longevity larder

BROCCOLI (CRUCIFEROUS VEGETABLES)

Broccoli was first cultivated in Italy over 2,000 years ago. It is part of the cruciferous family of vegetables, which includes cauliflower, kale, cabbage, cavolo nero and Brussels sprouts. They all contain glucosinolates, which are sulphur-rich plant compounds that break down into their protective active compounds (like sulforaphane and indole-3-carbinol) when chopped or chewed. These compounds support liver-detoxification pathways, have anti-inflammatory effects, and may help regulate cellular-defence mechanisms. Sulforaphane metabolizes to glutathione, a major antioxidant in the body. Broccoli is also a source of indole-3-carbinol, which supports oestrogen detoxification too. Freeze-dried broccoli sprouts contain a lot of sulforaphane and can be added to soups, salads and stews for extra antioxidant support.

blood pressure

Black and South Asian women in the UK may be up to three or four times more likely to suffer from high blood pressure than the rest of the population. There are many reasons cited for this, including socioeconomic and preventative-health disparities; genetics, such as renal salt sensitivity; and increased risk of type 2 diabetes in UK South Asian communities, which can lead to a risk of higher blood pressure. They can also experience higher levels of stress, resulting from sexism and racism – what is known as ‘psychological weathering’. These stats are just shocking and highlight not only medical sexism but medical racism, too. The DASH diet (Dietary Approaches to Stop Hypertension) was developed to help lower high blood pressure and reduce the risk of heart disease by focusing on vegetables, fruits, wholegrains, pulses, lean meat, nuts and seeds, and limiting salt, sugar, red meat and saturated fats. A high intake of vegetables gives us more potassium, which helps to dilate our blood vessels. Potassium works in partnership with sodium to regulate blood pressure: sodium constricts our blood vessels, while potassium dilates them. Potassium also helps lower blood pressure by getting rid of excess sodium, through the kidneys and out in the urine. I use herbs and spices to flavour my food; I only use salt sparingly in cooking, and don't add extra at the table. Plant-based foods are naturally low in salt – however, lots of ultra-processed plant-based products are often high in it. Vitamin D is really important for blood pressure too. Getting our 10,000 steps in each day is a great way of both staying active and getting some sunshine to increase our vitamin D, which research has shown can improve the pumping capacity of the heart.[56] Nitric oxide is a signalling molecule that helps maintain our vascular health. It is a vasodilator that relaxes and widens our blood vessels to increase blood flow and aid circulation as well as regulate blood pressure. It is also anti-inflammatory in nature, and has been shown to inhibit platelet aggregation (see p.66). Nitric oxide is also found in the gut, where it helps maintain adequate blood flow to the gut lining. As we age it can decline, but these foods can aid production: beetroot, celery, garlic, kale, spinach, watermelon, pomegranate and cacao. Stress is a huge factor, though, when it comes to blood pressure, but there are lots of tips on p.29 to help blunt its effects on the body. And as we saw in the Metabolic Harmony chapter, lows in blood sugar can also stimulate the stress response and vasoconstriction, which increases blood pressure. This is another cardiometabolic connection.

the importance of fibre for cholesterol removal

The focus for women wanting to lower cholesterol should be to help the body get rid of it efficiently – not to strip it all from their diet (although we don't want to be eating lots of high-cholesterol foods). Beneficial soluble fibre from plants helps with this process. When we eat high-fibre food, it stimulates the release of cholesterol-rich bile acids that are made in the liver and stored in the gallbladder. Foods high in fibre can reduce the reabsorption and recycling of these bile acids in the gut. The liver then draws on cholesterol in the blood to make more bile acids, thus reducing cholesterol levels. Beta glucans are soluble dietary fibres that form a gel-like substance when added to water. They are found in oats and barley. Numerous studies have shown that this kind of soluble fibre can lower LDL cholesterol levels and slow gastric emptying time. It's also a GLP-1 inducer. Just one serving of beans a day can lower LDL by 8 mg/dL,[57] and studies show that legume consumption can also reduce risk factors for cardiovascular disease.[58] Plant sterols are another important component of a fibre-rich diet. These are compounds found in plants that function in a similar way to cholesterol and are therefore thought to compete with cholesterol for absorption in the intestines, thereby reducing overall LDL levels. Various studies have also indicated that linseed oil may help reduce LDL levels.

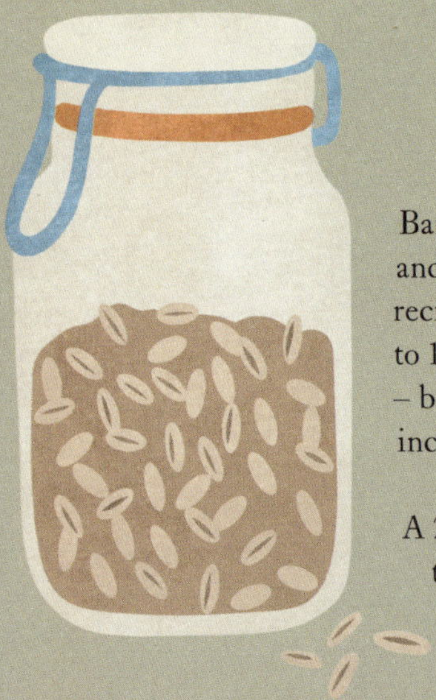

longevity larder

BARLEY (WHOLEGRAINS)

Barley has been cultivated for thousands of years, and may have been used for the very first recorded recipe for beer, found on a Sumerian tablet dating to 1800 BCE! It contains soluble fibre (beta glucan – between 3 and 11 per cent), which is thought to increase the excretion of bile acids.

A 2023 RCT crossover trial on oats and barley found that the regular consumption of both improved triglyceride and LDL cholesterol levels.[59]

movement

Movement is really important for our cardiovascular health, especially to build up the heart muscle and to lower blood pressure and support healthy blood vessels. However, if you are super stressed out, then HIIT is not what you need. Aim instead for lower intensity exercise and try to incorporate more mindful movement such as yoga and Pilates, alongside meditation and breathwork. Weight-bearing exercise will also still get your heart going and help to support your metabolic health, which is so key for cardiovascular health. Try to be more active during the day too – so many of us sit at a desk all day and then go for a 45-minute session in the gym and think that's us done. Some of the longest-living humans on the planet have never been to the gym! When I lived in Beijing, many elderly people would be doing tai chi in the park every day, or walking their tiny dogs, using the outdoor gym apparatus that was provided in most parks, or even doing ballroom-style dancing, which I loved to watch. They were active! There are many small things you can do to increase activity, such as always taking the stairs rather than the escalators. Try a stand-up desk, or if you are sitting for extended periods, make sure you get up regularly to move and stretch.

nutritional shifts:

* Cook with extra virgin olive oil and aim for unfiltered brands to increase the amount of polyphenols.
* Enjoy linseed oil in salad dressing, or consume one teaspoon a day.
* Aim for brightly coloured vegetables daily – beetroot, carrots and green leafy veg.
* Eat tomatoes for the antioxidant lycopene.
* Add garlic to your cooking (most of my recipes include it!)
* Eat oily fish two times a week (tinned is fine), such as salmon, sardines, mackerel, trout and herring.
* Prioritize quality protein sources for glycaemic control and essential amino acids for detoxification and methylation.
* Enjoy a thumb-sized portion of nuts a day, especially walnuts and almonds.
* Eat a daily portion of blueberries, pomegranate seeds, plums, green tea, cacao or beetroot for polyphenols and to aid production of nitric oxide.
* If you spend hours at a desk, increasing flavanol-rich foods such as cacao (see p.110 for why)
* Up turmeric and ginger in teas, tagines and curries.
* Eat organic soy three times a week (tofu, tempeh, miso, soya yogurt and edamame beans).
* Eat more oats and barley for soluble fibre.
* Eat more pulses, ideally daily, as they do in the Blue Zones – lentils, chickpeas, kidney and black beans and soya beans.
* Try this Ayurvedic remedy for reducing blood pressure: steep one stick of cinnamon, five cloves and a chunk of ginger in a cup of boiling water for five minutes or more. Drink and top up with extra boiled water throughout the day.

lifestyle shifts:

- Follow the stress-busting tips, including adaptogens, given on p.29 of the Metabolic Harmony chapter.
- Remember that meditation, yoga and breathwork will all help reduce stress and blood pressure.
- A lot of research has been carried out into the link between saunas and reduced blood pressure through vasodilation. They are also associated with reduced risk of sudden cardiac arrest and cardiovascular disease.[60]
- Cold-water immersion has been shown to be beneficial when it comes to lowering stress and inflammation. However, it is important to avoid it if you suffer from chronic stress, a heart condition or have blood-pressure issues because this therapy is an acute stressor, triggering an immediate response from the sympathetic nervous system.
- Exercise outside when you can for exposure to sunlight (and therefore for vitamin D) and to support mental well-being.
- Use a stand-up desk, or if you are sitting sit for long periods at a desk, take breaks for stretching.
- Alcohol is broken down and rebuilt into triglycerides and cholesterol in the liver – it basically raises your cholesterol levels. So keep your intake moderate and enjoy some of the many alcohol-free drinks now on the market, or simply have some days without it.

supplements to consider:

(Not to be taken all together and if you are on any medication, do speak to your healthcare practitioner first before starting any new supplements)

- Ancient + Brave, True Magnesium+
- Bare Biology, Life & Soul omega-3
- Bionutri, Cardiomega Plus
- BioCare, Female Balance (for phytoestrogens and polyphenols – not to be used if on HRT or with a history of breast cancer)
- Cytoplan, Organic Turmeric
- Invivo, Bio.Me Essential (for polyphenols)
- Linseed/flaxseed oil, one teaspoon a day

brain food

Our brain makes up around 2 to 3 per cent of our body weight and needs a whopping 20 to 25 per cent of our energy requirements! At menopause, our brains undergo a 'remodelling process', due in part to changes in oestrogen, which the brain is very sensitive to. The two other times that our brain will have undergone this process were during puberty and pregnancy. Baby brain is common postpartum due to changes in oestrogen, and the 'meno brain' is similar. Dr Roberta Brinton, a leading neuroscientist involved in research of the female brain, describes menopause as more of a neurological transition than a reproductive one. This chapter will do a deep dive into how we can support this neural reprogramming, to nourish our long-term cognitive health and reduce the risk of dementia and Alzheimer's.

Menopause is a time when the nerve cells (neurons) in our brain, are adjusting to not being reproductive. So that our brain can age well, we need to support this neural adaptation through our diet and lifestyle, both of which play vital roles in reducing risk. Cognitive changes are most evident in tests related to learning (encoding or processing information), recall of words (memory) and other verbal abilities,[61] and these changes begin at perimenopause. However, we must remember that all is not lost – the US multi-site Study of Women's Health Across the Nation (SWAN) shows that there is a cognitive bounce back post-menopause. A lot of longitudinal research has explored the ways that diet and lifestyle can reduce the risk of Alzehimer's risk and cognitive decline.[62] These include an anti-inflammatory, metabolically flexible, antioxidant-rich diet to protect against neuroinflammation and to remove toxins, as well as exercise, cognitive exercises and community.

oestrogen and the brain

Our brain is sensitive to changes in oestrogen. Two thirds of Alzheimer's patients are women and most of them are post-menopausal. A lot of women I speak to are worried that they are putting themselves at risk of dementia and Alzheimer's if they're not on HRT, especially if they have a parent with the condition, which I totally understand. At the moment, there is only data on women who have had an oophorectomy or surgical menopause benefiting from early HRT. If you haven't had a surgical menopause, there is no evidence to show that HRT provides a reduced

longitudinal research studies

The US Study to Protect Brain Health Through Lifestyle Intervention to Reduce Risk (US POINTER) was a clinical trial held over two years that showed that cognitive improvement in older adults at risk of cognitive decline and dementia, regardless of sex, ethnicity, genetic risk (APOE4 genotype) or heart health status.[63] Participants engaged in:

Physical exercise: 30 to 35 minutes of moderate-to-intense aerobic activity four times a week, plus strength and flexibility exercises twice a week.

Cognitive exercises: a computer-based brain-training programme three times a week for 30 minutes, plus regular engagement in other intellectually challenging and social activities.

Nutrition: the MIND diet, which emphasizes dark leafy greens, berries, nuts, wholegrains, olive oil and fish, and limits sugar and unhealthy fats.

The Finnish Geriatric Intervention Study to Prevent Cognitive Impairment and Disability (FINGER) is a double-blind, randomized controlled trial with 1,260 participants, aged 60 to 77. It has shown that lifestyle interventions can improve brain health and prevent cognitive decline[64] as well as cardiovascular risk.[65]

risk of dementia or Alzheimer's. Leading neuroscientist Dr Lisa Mosconi states that the evidence is all over the place at the moment, but is hopeful that her current research into women on HRT with biomarkers of Alzheimer's will change our understanding over the next few years. Diet and lifestyle shifts are crucial to mitigating our risk of cognitive decline. We do have agency over how our brain ages, regardless of whether we have lower oestrogen levels or the APOE4 genotype (although carrying this doesn't mean you are going to develop Alzheimer's).

Phytoestrogens can be really useful here as the brain gets used to lower levels. They are not oestrogen but exert a mild oestrogen-like effect on the body and brain and also have antioxidant qualities. The phytoestrogen found largely in soy is the isoflavone daidzein which is converted in the gut by intestinal flora to its metabolically active metabolite, equol. Studies have shown that dietary isoflavone intake is inversely associated with cardiovascular disease, cognitive decline and dementia in East Asian populations;[66] however, randomized controlled trials of soy isoflavones in Western countries did not show as much cognitive benefit. This discrepancy might be due to the fact that 40 to 70 per cent of East Asians produce equol from isoflavones, compared to 20 to 30 per cent of Westerners.[67] A pilot study into genistein, daidzein and equol in supplement form conducted by Dr Roberta Brinton et al, showed positive declines in hot flushes (due to the oestrogen-mimicking effect of phytoestrogens to buffer a dip in oestrogen, which can trigger a hot flush – more on these and the connection with our brain health later) as well as a reduction in cognitive decline.[68] More studies are needed, but increasing your phytoestrogen intake through food is such an important part of my menopause (and post-menopause) toolkit. These mild oestrogen-like, protective effects benefit not just for our nervous system but our cardiovascular and bone health too.

oestrogen, blood sugar and fuelling the brain

Oestrogen helps to increase glucose uptake into our cells due to a process called glycolysis, creating the body's energy currency ATP from glucose. Our brain's preferred fuel source is glucose but once reserves are depleted, our brain uses fat as a fuel source called ketone bodies, created in our mitochondria, when your body breaks down fat for energy. During menopause our brain has to adapt to using ketone bodies as an alternative fuel when glucose is in short supply.[69] We have thousands to millions of mitochondria in each neuron because our brain is energy-hungry, so any out-of-balance fuel supply has a massive impact on our cognition. This is why it is so important to reduce high carbohydrates foods post-menopause (well, at any time really), and as discussed in the Metabolic Harmony chapter – being able to switch between fuel sources is essential. This is yet another sign of the way that our metabolic health affects our nervous system. Beta-hydroxybutyrate (BHB) is the primary ketone produced during ketogenesis, which research suggests is particularly beneficial for conditions such as Alzheimer's.[70]

Lows in blood sugar cause the release of stress hormones adrenaline and noradrenaline, stimulating vasoconstriction, which increases blood pressure, and skin vasodilation, which can cause flushing. Supporting your blood sugar balance helps to support your cognition now and in the future (lows in blood sugar can make us feel irritable and we may also have trouble focusing); Dr Brinton and Dr Pauline Maki have both highlighted a connection between vasomotor symptoms of menopause and increases in cognitive impairment.[71] So, it's incredibly important to support balanced blood-sugar levels and metabolic flexibility so that ketones can be produced in the mitochondria for a steady energy supply within the brain.

reducing inflammation and oxidative stress

Often called neuroinflammation, inflammation and oxidative stress are two of the biggest drivers of cognitive decline, but thankfully, there is a lot of data on how our diet can help. As has been mentioned in previous chapters, antioxidants are incredibly important for dealing with the build-up of reactive oxygen species (ROS), which causes oxidative stress. Remember that ROS are produced post-ATP production in those thousands or sometimes millions of mitochondria (energy factories) we have in each of our brain cells. Build-up of DNA damage in our brain cells is linked to an increased risk of Alzheimer's and dementia. Increasing nutrients that support DNA repair (those SIRT and FOXO3 genes again) is incredibly important. For example, SIRT1 has been shown in numerous studies to be neuroprotective because it increases the breakdown of amyloid plaque.[72] Consuming a polyphenol-rich diet has a beneficial effect on modulating SIRT1. This includes: resveratrol (grapes, red wine, blueberries, cacao), quercetin (onion, kale, broccoli, apples, grapes), curcumin (turmeric), pterostilbene (berries, grapes, peanuts) and tetramethoxyflavone (found in the peel and pulp of citrus fruits).[73]

longevity larder

GREEN TEA

Originating in China, green tea is thought to have been enjoyed as a beverage for at least a thousand years. Coming from the *Camellia sinensis* plant, the most abundant antioxidant found in the tea is EGCG (epigallocatechin gallate), which is part of the catechin polyphenol family. EGCG is often noted in the scientific literature as having anti-inflammatory, neuroprotective, anti-tumour and cardioprotective properties.[74] Green tea also contains L-theanine, which helps to support GABA production, our overarching calming neurochemical, which is why it has been used for so long to aid relaxation.

Remember to not use boiling water, otherwise it can taste too bitter. Leave the kettle to stand for 5 to 10 minutes before pouring over the leaves.

One class of polyphenols that has a powerful anti-inflammatory effect on the brain are flavonoids. They include the compounds apigenin, resveratrol, catechins, rutin and curcumin, and are found in globe artichokes, basil, berries, buckwheat, celery, citrus fruits, green tea, parsley, red grapes and turmeric. Vitamins C and E also have antioxidant properties and are hugely important for reducing oxidative damage in the brain. Oleuropein, a polyphenol found in extra virgin olive oil, has been shown in research to modulate PARP1 activation, which helps to protect nerve cells from oxidative damage. 8-OHdG is a marker for DNA damage, which increases with age particularly in those with Alzheimer's. Research has shown a reduction in this marker and reduced DNA damage for those who consumed 50 millilitres of extra virgin olive oil per day (that's around 3 tablespoons) for one year.[75] Pretty impressive! Not that you have to start downing olive oil shots – just incorporate it more into your food by using it as your main cooking oil, as well as in pesto, salsa verde, salad dressings or swirled on top of soups.

As we know, inflammation and neuroinflammation can be components of the menopausal transition, but there are many foods that can help. Nuts, and especially walnuts, are high in omega-3 essential fatty acids, which exert an anti-inflammatory effect on the brain. Both walnuts and almonds are also high in antioxidant-rich vitamin E and flavonoids that protect the blood–brain barrier (flavonoids are particularly concentrated in the nuts' wispy outer skins). They are also full of the fibre essential for our second brain, the gut. One study relates to data from the Harvard Nurses' Health Study, for which 50,000 women were followed for more than two decades in an observational trial.[76] Those who ate five or more servings of nuts per week had better cognitive scores later in life, and they scored as if they were two years younger. The PREDIMED trial in Spain showed that older adults at higher CVD risk who followed the Mediterranean diet enriched with nuts had significantly better cognition and memory after just four years than those on a standard low-fat diet.[77]

The essential omega-3 fats are important for brain function and a healthy nervous system. They keep the neuron's membrane healthy, enabling brain cells to communicate with one another. They are also important (alongside other fats including EVOO) for aiding the absorption of fat-soluble vitamins A, D, E and K. Deficiencies in these nutrients can have a profound effect on brain health; for example, a lack of vitamin D is associated with increased inflammation and accelerated brain ageing.[78]

longevity larder

TURMERIC

What can turmeric not do? Curcumin is the polyphenol found in the turmeric root. It comes up in research time and again (with over 41,000 research papers to date!) due to its potent anti-inflammatory, analgesic and antioxidant properties, and has been used for healing systems by different cultures for millennia. It is also rich in iron, manganese, potassium and vitamin C. New studies show links between turmeric and improvement of blood glucose control, cardiovascular disease and depression, as well as possible anti-cancer mechanisms. Buy fresh if you can, which lasts for ages, although be wary of yellow fingers when prepping it! Increase its absorption by eating it with fat sources or with piperine from black pepper.

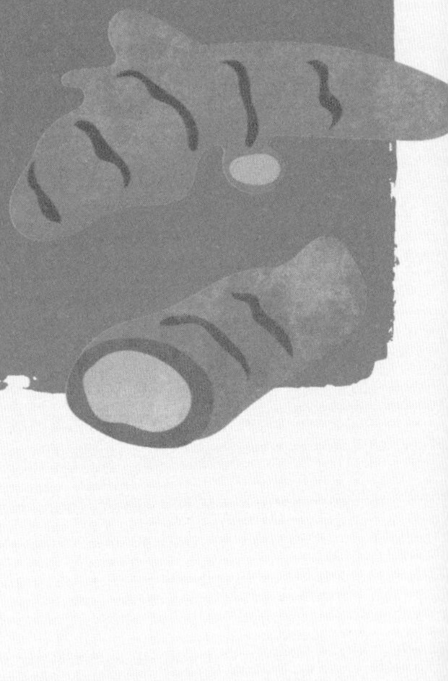

other key nutrients

Studies have shown legume consumption can have a positive effect on cognition performance in the elderly.[79] Additional cognitive decline protection was seen in research where participants swapped 5 per cent of animal protein for plant protein sources from beans and lentils.[80] The Nurses' Health Study and the Health Professionals Follow-Up Study both found a 26 per cent lower risk of cognitive decline when people swapped animal protein for plant proteins like beans.[81] A good case for more beans in your diet!

Some important herbs and spices include sage, lemon balm, saffron, turmeric and rosemary (see p.86). Sage helps slow the breakdown of a key brain chemical called acetylcholine, which is important for memory, concentration and focus. It has been shown to have a positive effect on Alzheimer's patients too. Lemon balm has been shown to reduce the breakdown of the memory transmitter acetylcholine. Saffron has antioxidant and neuroendocrine and neuroprotective qualities. It may reduce beta-amyloid-induced neuronal apoptosis (the build-up of plaques) and improve cognitive function in Alzheimer's. It helps to increase antioxidant levels in the hippocampus, which can then reduce memory impairment. Many studies have suggested that curcumin from turmeric may be an effective therapy for Alzheimer's because it exerts neuroprotective actions through numerous pathways, including antioxidant activity. It's known to reduce amyloid plaque formation and can cross the blood brain barrier to reduce inflammation.[82]

Choline is found in eggs and is an important part of acetylcholine, as well as phosphatidylcholine. It can improve cognition in mild to moderate Alzheimer's patients.

As mentioned previously (see p.16), gut dysbiosis is one of the hallmarks of ageing. This can have a massive impact on how our brain ages too, due to changes in the absorption of nutrients in the gut, metabolism and the arrival of nutrients and polyphenols through the blood–brain barrier to help control brain inflammation and oxidative stress. The brain does not like toxins! Fibre is so incredibly important for supporting our beneficial bacteria, as it is for all of the other aspects of health covered in this book. You should be aiming for 30 grams of fibre daily, and the foods that I recommend – as well as the recipes provided – will deliver that easily.

Brain-derived neurotrophic factor (BDNF) is linked to better cognitive function – it is basically food for your brain cells. It supports the survival of brain cells and encourages the growth of new ones. It plays a critical role in brain plasticity, to help support memory storage. Reduced levels are seen in normal ageing but also conditions such as Huntington's, Alzheimer's and Parkinson's disease.[83] Exercise increases BDNF levels, and vitamin D and omega-3 fatty acids have been shown to increase levels too.[84] Exercise outside! People with lower levels of vitamin D have a greater risk of experiencing substantial cognitive decline.[85] Fasting has

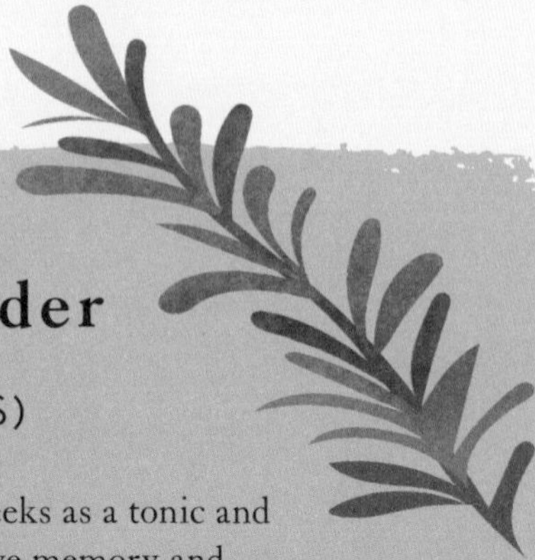

longevity larder

ROSEMARY (HERBS)

This herb was traditionally used by the ancient Greeks as a tonic and stimulant to strengthen mental function and improve memory and concentration, and students would wear crowns of rosemary during exams for this reason. Modern-day research shows that this cognitive improvement might be due to rosemary's polyphenol, rosemarinic acid, which may protect brain cells and preserve the memory neurotransmitter acetylcholine, along with antioxidants such as carnosic acid, which protects against oxidative stress linked to cognitive decline. Hence the expression 'rosemary for remembrance'.

kashmiri tea

I was lucky enough to drink this tea in Srinagar in Kashmir, near to all the saffron fields.

MAKES 1 CUP

A pinch of saffron
2 almonds, halved

Put the saffron and almonds into a cup and add just-boiled water and leave to steep to let the saffron diffuse for a few minutes.

also been shown to increase BDNF. Studies have shown that intermittent fasting can result in metabolic stress, which stimulates the production of proteins involved in synaptic plasticity, the building of new brain cells (neurogenesis), neuronal survival, memory and learning.[86] There's no need to do those crazy three-day fasts you might have heard of – most of this research is based on the 16:8 fasting schedule, where the brain is more likely to switch to burning fat (ketones). However, time-restricted eating for 10 hours with a 14-hour overnight fast (which is what I do) will still be beneficial, and for insulin sensitivity and cellular repair, too.

Homocysteine is a naturally occurring amino acid produced as part of the body's methylation process (a biochemical process that occurs in the body billions of times a second; see pp. 18–19). Folate, B12 and B6 are incredibly important for this process. Elevated levels of homocysteine are known to be a risk factor for cardiovascular disease (see the Queen of Hearts chapter) but have also been shown to correlate with cognitive decline. Even though folate, B12 and B6 can help homocysteine stay within normal range, there are numerous other factors at play when it comes to elevated levels, such as medications, genetic variations, smoking, alcohol, advancing age and obesity.

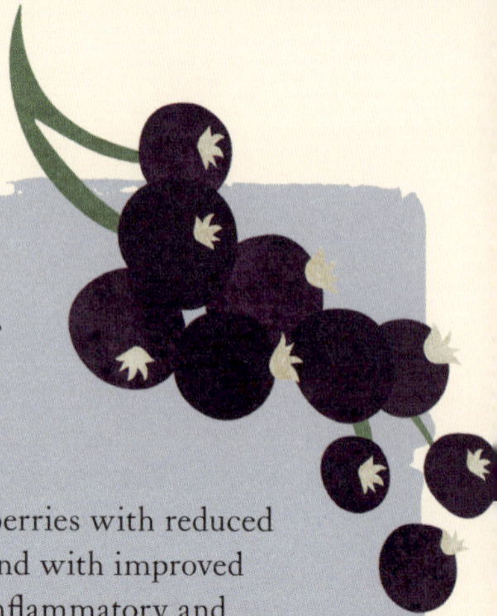

longevity larder

BERRIES & CHERRIES

Studies have associated a regular, moderate intake of blueberries with reduced risk of cardiovascular disease, type 2 diabetes and death, and with improved weight maintenance and neuroprotection too.[87] The anti-inflammatory and antioxidant effects of pomegranates have also been well researched, delivering nearly 30 milligrams of vitamin C (UK RDA is 40 milligrams) and polyphenols such as anthocyanidins and ellagic acid. Cherries are high in vitamin C and K, copper and manganese, and polyphenols including beta carotene, lutein, zeaxanthin, anthocyanins, quercetin, chlorogenic acid, ellagic acid and gallic acid. The Romans introduced the first cherry trees to Britain from Persia. It is thought that you can trace old Roman roads in Britain by the wild cherry trees – the Roman legions spat out stones from the fruit as they travelled the country.

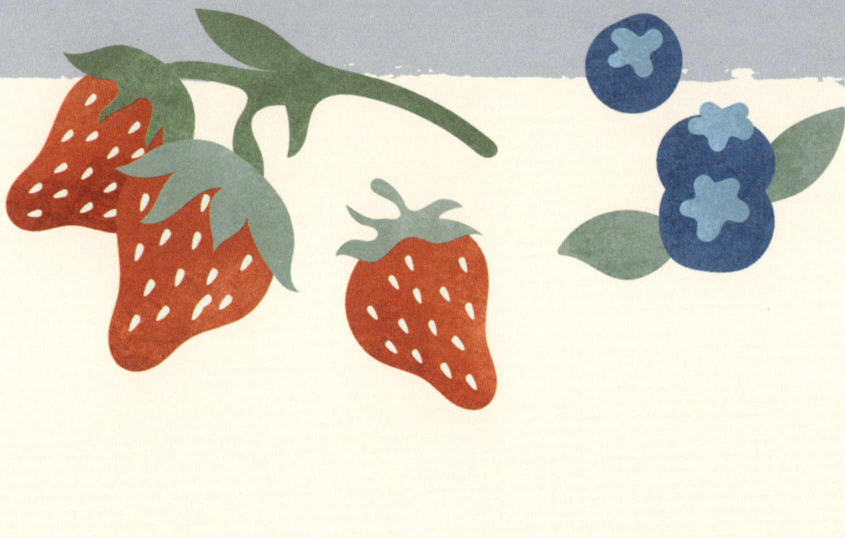

nutritional shifts:

- Use extra virgin olive oil for salad dressings, pesto, salsa verde and in all your cooking.
- Eat oily fish at least two to three times a week and enjoy linseed oil as a plant-based additional source of omega-3 fats and vitamin E.
- Enjoy nuts and seeds daily.
- Eat your greens daily! For folate, iron, and vitamin C and K.
- Eat B12-rich foods: meat, fish, dairy and fortified plant-based foods.
- Enjoy a handful of berries daily.
- Enjoy plenty of herbs, especially rosemary and sage.
- Up your spices, especially saffron and turmeric.
- Add in more phytoestrogen-rich plants: tofu, tempeh, soya, linseed/ flaxseed, alfalfa, pulses, beans, peas, chickpeas, broccoli and cabbage, sage and red clover.
- Eat eggs for choline. Choline is essential for making acetylcholine, the memory neurotransmitter.
- Phenylalanine converts to tyrosine for alertness, attention and focus: sources include pumpkin seeds, Parmesan, soya beans, lean beef, chicken, salmon, mackerel, cod, eggs and pinto beans.
- L-theanine is an amino acid found in green tea (opt for decaf) that is traditionally used to enhance relaxation and improve concentration. It also supports SIRT1.
- Avoid refined sugar where possible, as well as fried and processed foods.
- Include coconut oil for cooking as a source of medium-chain tryglycerides (MCTs), which support ketogenesis.
- Get outside more often for vitamin D, and take a vitamin D supplement.
- Reduce toxin exposure where possible, such as exhaust fumes, cigarette smoke, pollution, plastics, solvents, cling film and aluminium foil.

lifestyle shifts:

Exercise is hugely important for reducing our risk of cognitive decline. It creates brain-derived neurotrophic factor; it is basically brain food. Exercise also helps us to be more sensitive to insulin, which improves blood-sugar balance and helps support improved communication by building new networks in the brain. It is also a brilliant de-stressor and anxiety buster!

Cognitive reserve is a term used to refer to the brain's ability to withstand the damage that comes with ageing or neurological diseases, and to continue to function optimally. This is what I hope this chapter will help you with. A study on nuns that began in the 1980s[88] suggests how to optimize our cognitive reserve. This was a longitudinal study of ageing and dementia on a cohort of 678 nuns across the US. All of the nuns agreed to donate their brains to medical science post-mortem, too. Their brains were shown to have a high cognitive reserve, which might've been due to their lifelong education, social interaction, emotional well-being, staying active and living with purpose. Keeping our brain active also helps us to maintain cognitive function and resilience, despite the consequences of ageing. Menopause can be the start of learning something new – taking on that idea of lifelong learning, by finding some new hobbies and areas of interest. The more we learn, the more synaptic connections we make, which can lead to greater brain plasticity.

Sleep is hugely associated with our cognitive health. It is essential for the release of cerebrospinal fluid, which acts a bit like a dishwasher on the brain, helping to clear toxins and amyloid plaques, which are associated with Alzheimer's disease. Research suggests that sleeping fewer than six hours may increase the risk of Alzeihmer's.[89] I know this might be distressing to hear if you are someone who suffers with sleep issues – there's nothing worse than being told you have to prioritize sleep if you can't get to sleep! I often think the term 'sleepmaxxing', which is used a lot now, can make us even more anxious about getting a good night's sleep. Some super-simple interventions you can start with include going to bed at the same time every day, drinking less (or no) caffeine, avoiding alcohol, not eating too late in the evening (the heat from digestion can affect our sleep), and eating more magnesium-rich foods, including in glycinate form as a supplement with your evening meal. Magnesium chloride baths are also a nice way to relax if you get wired and tired. Avoid foods high in tyramine and histamine in the evening, which can increase adrenaline and stop us sleeping – cheese, wine and cured meats, for example. Getting early morning light also helps to nourish our circadian rhythm, our sleep–wake cycle, and using blue-light blocking glasses in the evening can help tell our body and brain that it is nearly bedtime. Keep all phones out of the bedroom and stop scrolling an hour before bedtime! Even though your phone might be on airplane mode, your whole life is on that device, so best to move it to the hallway to charge.

supplements to consider:

(Not to be taken all together and if you are on any medication, do speak to your healthcare practitioner first before starting any new supplements)

- Bare Biology, Life & Soul omega-3
- Bare Biology, Vitamin D and K2
- BioCare, Female Balance (for phytoestrogens and antioxidants)
- BioCare, Vitamin D, 1000iu
- BioCare or Cytoplan, Magnesium Bisglycinate, to help support relaxation and sleep.
- Bristol Fungarium, Lion's Mane tincture. I have seen this help in my clinic – there was a small RCT trial done on this medicinal mushroom that showed benefits for cognition and memory.
- Cytoplan, Omega-3 Vegan
- Invivo, Bio.Me Essential (for polyphenols)
- The Linseed Farm, linseed oil. Not really a supplement but useful for salad dressings, or just take a teaspoon a day – keep it in the fridge.

unbreakable

FOODS TO SUPPORT OUR MUSCULOSKELETAL SYSTEM

This chapter is all about helping to support our musculoskeletal system post-menopause and reducing osteoporosis risk factors. We must remember that bone is a living, growing tissue, requiring nutrients and blood flow. Around 30 per cent of bone consists of an organic matrix, of which 90 per cent is collagen (mostly Type 1) and 70 per cent inorganic mineral component called hydroxyapatite. Together they form a flexible (collagen) and strong (minerals) framework so that our bones can withstand stressors and not fracture easily.

The word 'osteoporosis' is taken from the Greek *osteo*, meaning 'bone', and *poros*, meaning 'passage' or 'little hole'. It is known as a 'silent' disease, often only being diagnosed after a hip or wrist fracture. Declining oestrogen levels can mean that we start to lose bone mass more quickly around the menopause because oestrogen supports what is known as osteoblast activity – the formulation of new bone. Our bones are constantly breaking down and removing old or damaged bone using cells called osteoclasts, and renewing bone using cells called osteoblasts. This process is known as bone turnover – a constant and tightly regulated process that maintains our bone mass and skeletal homeostasis (balance). Our bone health is very sensitive to oestrogen but, as we will see in this chapter, there are many elements at play here, so we can do a lot through our diet and lifestyle to mitigate our risk.

The Royal Osteoporosis Society in the UK cites numerous factors that can increase our risk of osteoporosis, including our genes, ageing, being a woman, body frame size (smaller body frames can have a higher risk due to less of a bone 'bank' to draw on), lower nutrient intake (including calcium and vitamin D – and as an aside, we often hear about calcium and vitamin D being the nutrients associated with bone health, but there are at least 20 essential nutrients that we must get from our diet, including vitamins, minerals, amino acids and essential fats), smoking, a past eating disorder, excessive alcohol and a sedentary lifestyle. Please note that not being on HRT is not a risk factor. As you will see in this chapter, we have the agency to support our future bone health without HRT, and even if you are on HRT, all of these pointers will be important for when you come off it. The following are some additional risk factors:

- Low dietary calcium and other bone-building minerals and vitamins.
- Poor absorption of calcium
- Inflammation leading to cartilage and bone destruction
- Caffeine, sugar, red meat and carbonated drinks affect calcium absorption or can increase calcium excretion
- Lack of weight-bearing exercise
- Lack of sunshine

We do know that bone formation is highly sensitive to oestradiol. This does not mean we are going to get osteoporosis as there are many factors involved, but it can be exacerbated by lower levels. Phytoestrogens can be helpful – they are not oestrogen but they exert a mild oestrogen-like effect on the body. This is why phytoestrogens might help us, as our levels reduce post-menopause – sources include ground linseed/flaxseed, chickpeas, sprouted mung beans, fermented red clover, tofu, tempeh and edamame beans. Their phytoestrogenic benefits may prevent the loss of bone mineral content and reduce bone breakdown, although more research is needed.[90] An RCT trial on osteopenic post-menopausal women showed that genistein, the phytoestrogen found in soybeans, reduced bone loss after a one- and two-year period.[91]

protein and collagen

Protein makes up about 50 per cent of your bone volume and about one-third of its mass. Higher-protein diets have actually been associated with greater bone mass and fewer fractures when calcium intake is adequate.[92] Amino acids build collagen, which is the scaffold that minerals attach to. Insulin-like growth factor 1 (IGF-1) is stimulated by higher protein intake, which is needed to stimulate bone growth (important in young women, too, who haven't achieved peak bone mass yet). This is why quality protein intake is essential for our bone mass at midlife. Collagen is the most abundant protein in the body. It's also important to note that we can lose up to 30 per cent of our collagen during menopause, which is a key component of bone and cartilage, and is why osteoarthritis can also be a common issue at this time. There are many different types of collagen but these are the main ones: Type I is abundant in all tissues, but is mostly concentrated in bones, skin and tendons. Type II is the main component of cartilage. Type III is found in soft tissue such as blood vessels and skin. Bone broth is an excellent source of collagen and easy to digest, so start making your own after a roast. Eggs, lean red meat, fish and poultry are also sources. There is no such thing as vegan collagen. Instead you need to increase the building blocks that support collagen synthesis in the body, which include glycine-rich tofu, nuts, and seeds, and proline-rich alfalfa sprouts, asparagus, beans, buckwheat, cabbage, cucumber and tempeh, along with vitamin C, zinc, biotin and copper. Studies have shown that collagen peptide supplementation might increase bone mineral density alongside vitamin D and calcium supplementation.[93]

calcium and other nutrients

There's a lot more to bone health than just calcium! It doesn't work in isolation to strengthen your bones. The architecture of bone requires many nutrients to maintain and restore its integrity, such as calcium, magnesium, manganese, zinc, phosphorous, boron, copper, amino acids and collagen, essential fatty acids EPA and DHA, isoflavones (from tofu, tempeh, miso and edamame), antioxidants such as lycopene (high in tomatoes) and vitamins A, B6, B9 (folate), B12, C, D and K.

Disturbances in calcium metabolism are a key factor in the development of osteoporosis because more than 99 per cent of the body's calcium is contained in the bones and teeth. Calcium has a synergistic relationship with other nutrients like vitamin K, vitamin D and magnesium.[94] There are two main types of vitamin K – K1 or phylloquinone is the main type, found in green leafy vegetables, and K2, known as menaquinone, which is produced by our gut bacteria. Vitamin K is needed for blood clotting as well as healthy bones. It helps to get calcium to the teeth and bones by activating a protein called osteocalcin, so you might have enough calcium but without adequate vitamin K then you might not get it to all of the places it's needed. A report from the Nurses' Health Study suggests that women who get at least 110 micrograms of vitamin K a day are 30 per cent less likely to break a hip than women who get less than that.[95] A review of six studies with over 93,000 participants suggested a decrease in fracture risk with higher vitamin K consumption.[96] Data from a longitudinal study, the NHANES study, showed an association between medium to high vitamin K intake in women and a reduced risk of osteoporosis.[97]

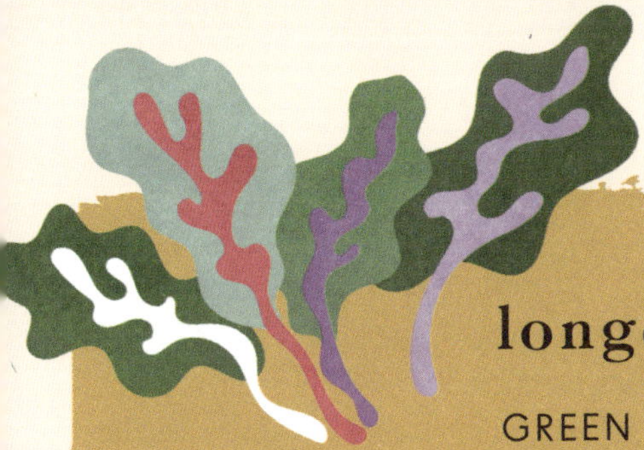

longevity larder

GREEN LEAFY VEGETABLES

Eat your greens…for your brain, your bones and your heart. These vegetables need to be on our plate daily – especially spinach, watercress, kale, cavolo nero, chard and spring greens. Watercress is one of the oldest greens recorded, used by the ancient Greeks, who considered it a valuable brain food and believed it strengthened the nervous system. A recent study showed that consuming just one serving per day of green leafy vegetables may help to slow cognitive decline, due to the nutrients that are found in large quantities in green leafy vegetables including folate, vitamin K and vitamin E, as well as antioxidants phylloquinone, lutein and kaempferol.[99]

Vitamin D is also crucial – without sufficient amounts, your body can only absorb around 10 to 15 per cent of your dietary calcium.[98]

Eating foods that contain an abundance of calcium alongside magnesium and vitamin K is therefore hugely beneficial, and I do recommend a vitamin D supplement all year round. Dairy sources contain the most calcium, but even though they are helpful providers of the mineral, they don't deliver so many of the co-factors for its absorption. Green leafy vegetables, for example, will deliver calcium, magnesium and vitamin K AND help to feed the beneficial bacteria in the gut to convert it to K2 to aid absorption too. Isn't mother nature clever?

inflammation and our bones

As with many other things, when it comes to our bones, the components that make up the Mediterranean diet are very helpful – for example, extra virgin olive oil, which may help to prevent bone pathology[100] due to its phenolic (polyphenol) content. The diet is also naturally high in polyphenols and omega-3s, which help to keep inflammation and oxidative stress down to support bone integrity.[101]

Inflammation in the body can be triggered by a diet that is high in ultra-processed foods, an unhealthy gut, excess fat around the middle, autoimmune conditions and even gum disease. A large review in 2025 showed that inflammatory markers are linked with increased risk of osteoporosis.[102] This is why there is positive research on bone health and anti-inflammatory omega-3 essential fatty acids eicosapentaenoic acid (EPA) and docosahexaenoic acid (DHA).[103] They are found in the highest quantities as EPA and DHA in oily fish, and in plant sources like algae, often in supplement form. Other anti-inflammatory foods include plenty

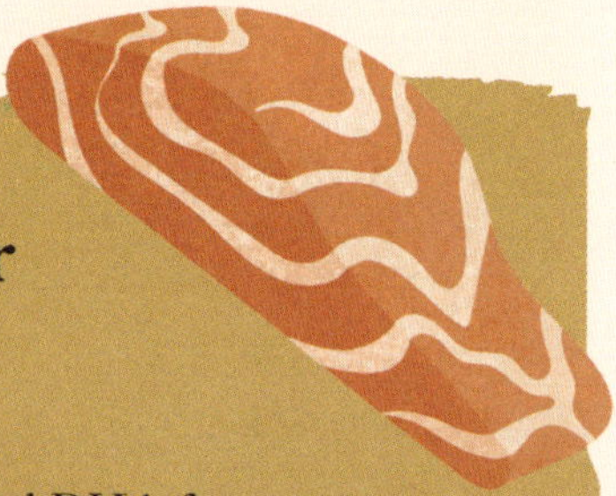

longevity larder

OILY FISH

Oily fish is the best source of omega-3 fats in their EPA and DHA form, which exert an anti-inflammatory effect on the body and brain. There is a great deal of research demonstrating their benefits for our mental well-being, our cardiovascular health and our bones. Omega-3 was first discovered by Danish scientists studying the Greenland Inuit, due to their low instances of cardiovascular disease and high intake of oily fish. Oily fish are also great sources of protein, B vitamins, vitamin D (found mostly in the skin) and calcium (especially sardine bones). I would opt for smaller fish to reduce levels of heavy metals like mercury, such as salmon, sardines, herring, mackerel and trout. Linseeds/flaxseeds and their oil, hemp oil and nuts (particularly walnuts) are vegan sources of omega-3 and need to be converted from alpha-linolenic acid to EPA and DHA. And, as mentioned earlier, you can also get vegan EPA and DHA sources of omega-3 from algae, usually in supplement form.

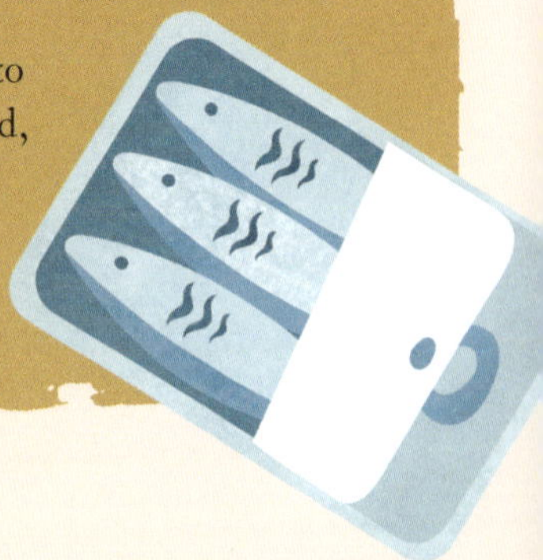

of leafy greens, berries, fermented foods, and herbs and spices – parsley, thyme, rosemary, turmeric and ginger – which should be accompanied by a reduction in more pro-inflammatory foods, such as fizzy drinks, alcohol, refined foods, sugar, excess salt and caffeine, which can all affect inflammation and bone turnover.

the gut–bone axis

The Mediterranean diet is also high in fibre, as with most traditional diets around the world, which is essential for a well-functioning gut and the production of short-chain fatty acids (SCFA). Butyrate, the most

longevity larder

FERMENTS

Fermenting is an ancient practice, beer having been brewed since the 6th millennium BCE by peoples living in Mesopotamia, ancient China and Egypt. Evidence of what is thought to be the earliest evidence of winemaking comes from Georgia, dating to around 6000 BCE. Fermentation was likely first discovered by accident, when yeasts and bacteria transformed stored foods such as milk and grains. Kimchi was being made by the 13th century using radishes rather than cabbage, and the term sauerkraut was being used in Germany in the 16th century. Fermentation was used primarily for food preservation over the winter. Now we know about the beneficial bacteria that are contained within them, in addition to other nutrients – making sauerkraut with cabbage can increase the vitamin C content by up to 50 per cent! It is best not to cook fermented foods as that destroys the beneficial bacteria. Just add miso or sauerkraut or kefir or kimchi to warm as opposed to super-hot dishes.

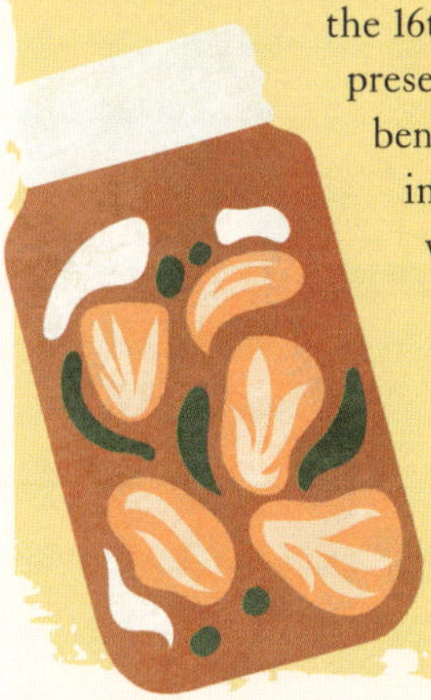

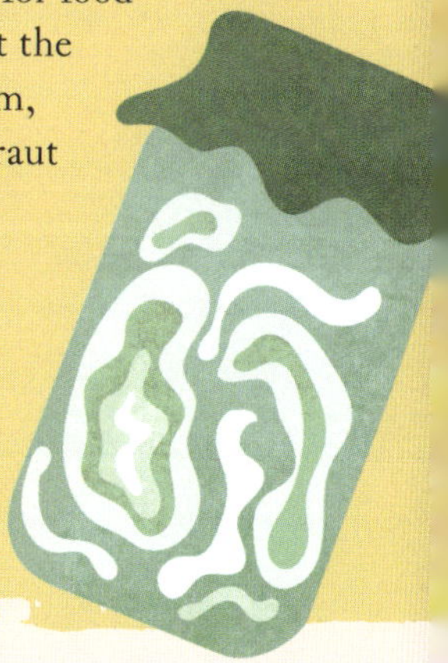

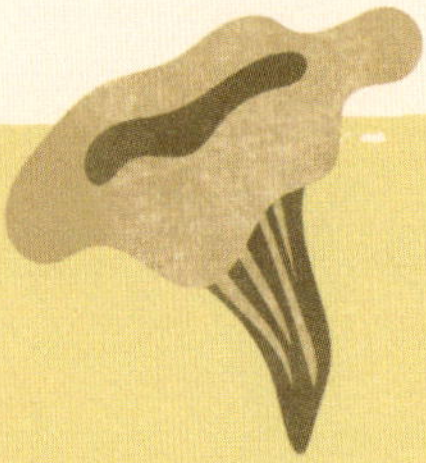

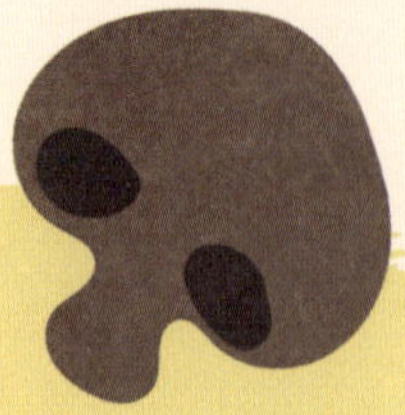

the longevity larder

MUSHROOMS

Mushrooms are a good source of copper for our nervous system, beta glucans for our gut, and vitamin D, if they have been grown under UV lights. Mushrooms are the best source of dietary ergothioneine, a potent antioxidant that protects cells from oxidative stress and inflammation – porcini, oyster and shiitake mushrooms having the highest concentrations. Medicinal mushrooms – used for more than 2,000 years in Traditional Chinese Medicine – such as cordyceps and reishi are also classified as adaptogens, to help us when stress levels are high. And a small RCT trial recently showed that lion's mane may support memory and cognition (although this was in young adults, so more research is needed).[104] However, it's great to see that modern science may be catching up with ancient remedies.

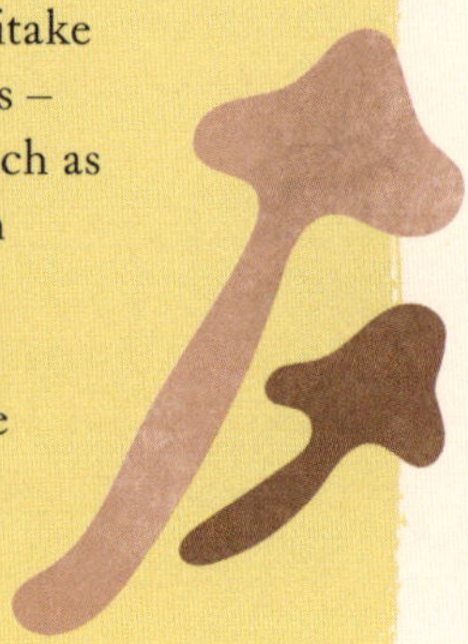

abundant SCFA, has been shown to stimulate bone formation, and other SCFAs also have direct effects on bone metabolism and its homeostasis.[105] We have to see our gut as being a key part of our bone health – without good gut function, calcium, as well as all the other essential bone nutrients, won't be absorbed as well and the gut bacteria won't produce vitamin K2 or SCFAs efficiently. This is known as the gut–bone axis.

MENOPAUSE, MIDLIFE AND MUSCULOSKELETAL HEALTH – WHAT WE NEED TO KNOW

Dinah Siman
Author, Yoga and Pilates Teacher

Have you heard of the term the 'musculoskeletal syndrome of menopause'? Don't worry, you're not alone, it's relatively new and I think it's a good new term for our meno vocab. It sounds scary because it's a 'syndrome', which always rings worry bells, but actually it's a recognition that menopause impacts our muscles, bones, joints, connective tissue, collagen, ligaments, tendons, fascia and any tissue in our feeling body. This highlighting of the physical pain that oestrogen depletion can cause is a positive step – it increases our own awareness and that of all healthcare professionals to the need to have musculoskeletal health on the radar – before, during and post-menopause. Muscle has been described as the organ of longevity. In simple terms, the more muscle we have, the longer we can get out of a chair, off the loo and take care of ourselves. There's a medical term, 'sarcopenia', which pops up as we age. It means the loss of muscle mass and the subsequent loss of movement ability. Now there's also the term 'osteosarcopenia', which chunks in the loss of bone density into the mix. It all sounds rather grim, I know, but it really doesn't have to feel like that at all. Spin it around and let's consider what this information gives us: empowerment. I truly believe midlife and menopause give us another opportunity to reassess just what we are doing for ourselves, where we are heading and how we can absolutely thrive in the next phases of life.

Undoubtedly knowledge gives personal power, and we are so fortunate in these times to have access to research, evidence and inspiration to support us in our choices. We can be informed, we can find the best ways to support our midlife body. Taking a good critical look at our musculoskeletal health can be informative, transformative and a lot of fun – it's not all doom and gloom!

Where to start – here's the thing. What do you enjoy? Have you been a gym bunny, a runner, aerobics fan, or are you loving your Pilates or yoga? Maybe you hate all exercise – I have plenty of clients who do, you're not alone, and all is not lost. We have to understand why appropriate movement practice matters, how we can benefit and then find the fit for us individually.

Muscle strength is vital for everyday living. We all know that hauling a load of shopping out of the car, moving plant pots, shifting furniture and picking up children demands strength. That muscle strength is also key to supporting our joints and our bones. There's a big trend for 'lifting heavy' at the moment, and that is admirable, but can feel intimidating. So, let's figure this out.

What does my body need?

- Cardio for heart strength and health
- Strength training for muscle mass
- Load for bone health
- Balance, co-ordination, fascial recoil, core strength, mobility, flexibility – for every body-wide system, including muscle strength and bone loading

That seems like a lot, I know, but we start where we are.

What if you have injuries? What if you're out of condition to start?

What if you're very tired? No time? Hate exercise? Too expensive?

Pause. Take a breath and let's plan.

Begin with walking. It's free, it's our natural movement and it supports our body and mind – win–win! If you love it, then add in a wrist hand weight or a small backpack with water bottles in to increase the challenge, up your heart rate and feel the progress.

Too much pain? Try Pilates to start. This is a very safe way to navigate your journey back to movement. As you gain confidence and trust your body, you can add in resistance with weights and bands, and you learn solid technique to take with you to any other exercise method.

Exercising with a friend is a great way to keep motivated; accountability is a great help for focus. Go to a class together, keep each other on track.

The idea of lifting weights can feel difficult, challenging and unfamiliar. It was new to me! But I have grown to love it. It's a super-efficient way to get my cardio exercise in and work on muscle mass in one hit – win–win in my book. I confess, I hate cardio. I know, I'm in the fitness industry, but in truth I've never liked it. Now, lifting weights I can benefit from cardio and increased strength and in a shorter time – what's not to love?! If it's a new concept to you then check out your local fitness centre and see if they offer an introduction to lifting weights. Or if you have any injuries but want to pursue lifting, check in with a healthcare professional like a physiotherapist for advice on the best route for you. Small steps lead to big wins in the long run.

Nutrition and movement are both key to ageing positively. We have the ability to influence how our body responds to menopause and beyond by our choices. Looking to improve our muscle strength and believing it's possible by doing it and feeling the results is really important. Don't take my word for it, try it. Trust your experience.

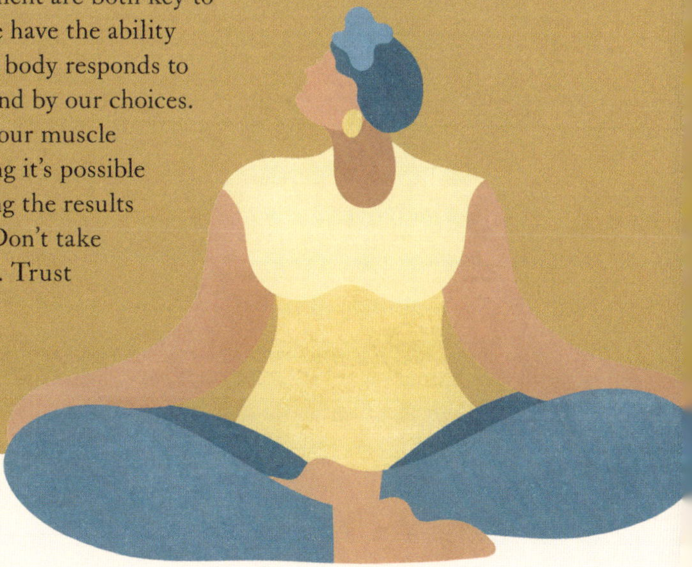

nutritional shifts:

- To get a good supply of calcium and co-factor foods (sources of magnesium and vitamin K too) eat green leafy vegetables daily: kale, spinach, cabbage, broccoli, pak choi and watercress.
- Include dairy sources of calcium, such as Greek yogurt, organic natural yogurt, cheese, cottage cheese and kefir.
- Enjoy non-dairy calcium sources too: tahini, tofu, tempeh, almonds, Brazil nuts, organic soya yogurt and sardines (the little bones are an added source).
- Enjoy more fermented foods to support your beneficial gut bacteria as well as vitamin K2 absorption (particularly natto and sauerkraut).
- Get your daily dose of Vitamin D, which is best absorbed from the sun and in supplement form. You will find some in mushrooms grown under UV lights and oily fish skin.
- Enjoy more protein-rich foods at every meal (three times a day). Start your day with eggs or scrambled tofu, or porridge with plenty of nuts and seeds and nut butter, or Greek yogurt with a high-protein granola, again with lots of nuts and seeds.
- Consume more collagen-rich foods, such as fish, eggs, poultry, red meat and bone broth (pop your chicken carcass in a pressure cooker and make your own).
- Alternatively, seek out vegan sources of collagen building-blocks: glycine-rich tofu, nuts and seeds, and proline-rich alfalfa sprouts, asparagus, beans, buckwheat, cabbage, cucumber and tempeh. Remember to get adequate vitamin C to support collagen synthesis.
- Drink nettle tea (which is high in calcium!).
- Up your anti-inflammatory omega-3 oils from oily fish twice a week with trout, salmon, mackerel, herring or sardines (tinned are fine!). Vegan omega-3 can be found in linseed/flaxseed oil (not to be heated).
- Add turmeric – lots of recipes are included in this book.
- Add ginger – again, found in lots of the recipes in this book! Grate it onto porridge or add a slice to hot water with a cinnamon stick or a slice of lemon.
- Aim for a handful of berries a day – blueberries, blackcurrants, blackberries and pomegranates (frozen are also fine).

lifestyle shifts:

Start doing weight-bearing exercise and work up to three times a week. You will build up your weights in no time! Online platforms are really helpful, especially for us time-poor women! I like Davina McCall's Own Your Goals (lots of beginner programmes on there), Kate Rowe-Ham's Owning Your Menopause and Caroline's Circuits.

Exercise outside if you can, to get your dose of vitamin D – run, hike, walk, play tennis, do a park run or a park boot camp, swim in the sea or at a lido (I'm lucky enough to have one nearby).

supplements to consider:

(Not to be taken all together, and if you are on any medication, do speak to your healthcare practitioner before starting any new supplements)

All of these supplements steer clear of calcium carbonate, which is basically chalk, and requires higher levels of stomach acid to be absorbed. Calcium citrate and algae sources are better absorbed.

- Ancient + Brave, True Collagen
- Ancient + Brave, Noble Collagen (Type II, useful for cartilage support)
  Cytoplan, Bone Support
- Bare Biology, Beam & Balance, Vitamins D3 + K2 (both 100 mcg)
- Bare Biology, Pure Marine Collagen Powder
- BioCare, Vitamin D spray, 1000iu
- Bonebalance is a clinically studied and proven bioactive peptide collagen support[106]
- Correxiko, Marine Collagen Peptides Powder
- Together Health, Bone Aid (calcium derived from algae, which naturally is a source of vitamin K too)
- Wild Nutrition, Collagen 500 Plus
- WillPowders, Bovine Collagen

developing long-term longevity rituals

This chapter is all about striving for consistency over perfection and the benefits of movement and community, as well as having purpose and agency. It's about patterns of well-being as opposed to a rigid format of living, about finding connection with ourselves (and not constantly thinking of others), and emphasizing behaviours that have a positive influence on our health span post-menopause.

social nutrition

Let's start with the concept of social nutrition. Many communities around the world focus on food as nourishment and celebration, versus the deconstruction of food into its constituent parts (how much protein or carbs or fibre or calories or fat) that often happens in our modern-day world. Food should bring joy and connection, which I just don't see enough of. The Buddhist approach is to see food as meditation, with cooking teaching us patience, mindfulness and respect for ingredients. This includes being present in the moment, respecting the planet and making people happy. And during Ramadan, the ninth month of the Islamic calendar, community fasting ends with community feasting! Food becomes gratitude, centred around community. These approaches see food intertwined with community, connection and nourishment – much healthier than eating alone in front of a screen, or trying to control food intake, to eat 'perfectly', and feeling guilty when we don't.

eating close to nature

And what I mean here is eating real food, with minimal processing, as much as possible. Food is one of the strongest ties that we have to nature. I mean, we are also part of the natural world! Eating seasonally is a wonderful way to connect to the seasons more. Produce also tastes so much better when it's been picked in season and not flown halfway around the world. We are incredibly spoilt when it comes to our food choices and I think it's good to eat more seasonally, and not the same food all year round. This is so much more sustainable for the planet, too. And be in nature more. Numerous studies have found links between being in nature and an improved mood and increased life satisfaction.[107]

reducing xenoestrogens

We need to reduce xenoestrogens and other toxins in our food environment. We are often far too busy counting calories when we should be counting chemicals! Xenoestrogens are endocrine-disrupting chemicals that mimic oestrogen and can build up in our fat cells. Common sources of xenoestrogens include plastics (BPA), pesticides, cosmetics (parabens, phthalates), synthetic hormones and contaminated feed used in the meat and dairy industry. Remember that our skin is our biggest organ and absorbs chemicals from our beauty products and make-up, so it's important to look at the ingredients here too. I would also note to look at ingredients for intimate products, which should definitely be paraben-free. Here's how to reduce xenoestrogens:

- Make sure your cosmetics, shampoos, serums, moisturizers and fragrances don't contain phthalates and parabens. Choose natural or organic personal-care products instead – loads of great brands are now available.
- Buy organic when you can, especially meat and dairy.
- Avoid plastic containers and wrap – and if you do buy fruit and vegetables in this way, give them a good wash before eating. The amount of plastic used for fresh fruit and veg in supermarkets is outrageous!
- Don't store fatty foods in plastic – the xenoestrogens can migrate into the food. Put it into glass containers instead.
- Don't heat food in plastic.
- Environmental pollutants such as the forever chemicals polychlorinated biphenyls (PCBs) and dioxins have been identified as xenoestrogens. These pollutants are often found in contaminated water, soil and air.
- Increase your fibre intake to reduce absorption of xenoestrogens and microplastics.
- Eat more cruciferous vegetables and phytonutrients to help support xenoestrogen detoxification pathways.

everyday movement

Exercise and movement should be seen as part of your everyday longevity patterns. So many of us tend to sit at our desk all day, then think a 45-minute gym session is job done. The Blue Zones inhabitants don't go to the gym, but they move, walk, garden, and are not stuck at a desk for eight hours a day. Healthy muscle mass is so important for reducing frailty in later life, as well as the risk of insulin resistance, and muscles release myokines during exercise, which help modulate the immune system.

If you are desk-based, like I am a lot of the time, standing up regularly, stretching, and breaking up sitting time is the most important thing you can do. Two hours of uninterrupted sitting can be enough to make your blood vessels measurably less elastic. A 2025 RCT study (on just men, though, which is very annoying – why aren't trials now evenly sex-based?!) found that plant flavanols can help protect your arteries during long periods of sitting. Researchers gave healthy young men either a high-flavanol cocoa drink (around 700 milligrams) or a low-flavanol version.

longevity larder

CACAO

Cacao was the sacred drink of the Aztecs, related to Xochiquetzel, the goddess of fertility, and consumed only by nobility. It's always best to buy raw chocolate or cacao if you can. Cocoa that has been processed by alkalization (called the Dutch process – a process that neutralizes the acids, making the chocolate less bitter) can result in a much lower flavonoid content.

Cacao is rich in polyphenols, including catechins, proanthocyanidins and anthocyanidins. They support nitric oxide release, which has cardioprotective and anti-inflammatory effects.[108]

They then asked them to sit still for two hours. The low-flavanol group showed the usual decline in artery elasticity and blood flow. But the high-flavanol group didn't – their vessels stayed more responsive.[109] So enjoy more cacao-rich dark chocolate or hot chocolate along with some of the cacao-rich recipes found in this book!

How do we realistically factor more movement into our daily lives? My biggest bit of advice here is to do what you enjoy so that it doesn't feel like another drain on your already low bandwidth. Dancing around your kitchen to your favourite tunes played loudly can be excellent exercise. Take the stairs rather than the lift or the escalator, take a 20-minute brisk walk daily – walk for ten minutes and then turn around and try to get home quicker than that – walk with a friend for a catch-up, do an online strength session to save time, swimming is a great form of low-impact exercise (that will rarely result in injury), try yoga, Pilates, dance classes with a friend, day raves...and I can thoroughly recommend doing a Couch to 5k. These kinds of movement do not require punishment; they should be fun!

fostering a strong (female!) community

Okinawans create *moais* – groups of five friends who are committed to each other for life. I totally love this idea! I do often think that one of the most beautiful parts of ageing is the deep friendships it brings. The Harvard Study of Adult Development which is one of the longest-running studies to date (more than 80 years), revealed that close relationships, more than money or fame, are what keep people happy throughout their lives. A recent global report from the World Health Organization's Commission on Social Connection illustrated how strong social networks improve health and reduce risk of early death. Friendships increase endorphins, which reduce the activity of the hypothalamic–pituitary–adrenal axis that regulates the body's stress response. They also have impressive analgesic properties in the brain; endorphins are 20 to 30 times more powerful than morphine! Numerous studies have shown how positive relationships, along with helping others and volunteering, are associated with lower inflammatory markers such as IL-6 in middle age.[110]

oxytocin boosters

Oxytocin plays an important part in human bonding; it is released during childbirth to promote breastfeeding and is a key factor in the bond between mother and baby. It is also brought on by hugging – we all need to hug more! Cuddling, kissing, sex and masturbation all increase levels. A recent bit of research discussed the benefits of masturbation for relieving symptoms of menopause; especially for mood changes, as it helps to create feelings of relaxation and happiness, and has been found to help us get to sleep and stay asleep.[111] Listening to music, massage, stroking your dog or cat (they also get a boost!), spending time with friends and eating also stimulates the release of oxytocin.

feeling more *ikigai*

Another Japanese word that doesn't have a direct translation is *ikigai*, which means living a happy life with a healthy body and mind and a sense of purpose. It's about gaining that zest for life, however old you are, be that through seeing friends, your art, crafts, gardening or your work. A Japanese national survey conducted in 2018 found that 47.5 per cent of people aged 70 and older are active in ways including working, enjoying hobbies and participating in community activities. Crafting in midlife can reduce stress and provide a feeling of productivity too. Novel experiences activate neuroplasticity and new challenges boost dopamine – our motivation and joy molecule. Explore the unfamiliar!

nourishing our circadian rhythm

Our circadian rhythm (the body's natural 24-hour clock) is incredibly important for our physical and mental well-being and for restful sleep. More on sleep interventions in the Brain Food chapter, but I just wanted to add in here how important it is for us to connect with daylight, don't worry if you can't get outside first thing – how many of us have time to do that when we've just woken up and have millions of things to do? Although it might only take a couple of minutes, so do it if it works for you. Early morning and late afternoon are the best times for infrared (IF) light and near infrared (NIR) light. These longer wavelengths have been shown to benefit mitochondrial function and reduce oxidative stress.[112] Warm sand and rocks reflect IR and NIR wavelengths. Wood fires emit IR and NIR wavelengths, while saunas, although not emitting light, do emit far infrared radiation. It's also thought that wearing blue-blocking glasses in the evening can help tell the brain that it's nearly bedtime – blue light in our homes (from lighting and digital devices) can trick the body into thinking it's still daytime and thus raise cortisol. This is why we can often get a second wind! We need cortisol to reduce naturally in the evening so that melatonin can be released to bring on restful sleep. Eating at similar times of the day and going to bed at similar times also helps. Meditation can also help to calm a busy mind, and if you meditate in the morning, it allows you to set intentions for the day ahead. Small steps can make a big difference.

setting boundaries

Setting boundaries is really important for our mental well-being. I do think it is helpful to stop chasing those endless to-do lists, to start taking a lunch hour, and to stop agreeing to meetings at work over lunch or in the early evening. Burnout is real. Learning to say no is something I do with a flourish now I'm over 50! And instead, make time for movement, make home-cooked food and make time for cooking it too. Take the time, too, to weave in a supportive, gentle self-practice such as going to the sauna, cold-water swimming, meditation or breathwork. These all help us to feel more in the present moment. We need to focus on what it means to live well, not just about how long we can last. It focuses us on today – how are we going to care of ourselves today? How are we going to feed ourselves today? How are we going to set boundaries, so we don't burn out? How are we going to bring awareness to our self-nourishment? What are we going to let go of? I think when you reframe ageing as truly living and looking after ourselves more, it becomes a far more positive and nourishing experience.

HOW TO BE SELFISH: HOW TO HEAL YOUR RELATIONSHIP WITH YOURSELF AND START LIVING LIKE YOU MATTER TOO

Suzy Reading
Chartered Psychologist and author of *How to Be Selfish*

We've been raised to equate our self-worth with how little we need others, how selfless we are, and how well we keep all the other people happy all the time, but the competing pulls of midlife will have you inevitably questioning how possible, and if it is indeed possible, how sustainable all this self-denial is. Please can we give ourselves permission to fail at what's humanly impossible?

This will involve a courageous examination of the beliefs that keep us stuck in self-silencing. Every time guilt taps you on the shoulder or shame derails that nourishing gesture, ask yourself why? What is the underlying belief? Hold it up to the light and ask whether you hold other people to account in the same way? Would you want your daughter, your son, or your best friend to adhere to this belief? Reflect on your values and allow them to also include you. That's not a transgression but a more honest and complete expression of them.

Let's take a closer look at selflessness. In moments, it might be possible, but we know it is not tenable long term. Pause to reflect on the consequences of you ignoring or dismissing your needs and feelings. Do this long enough and you will wind up burnt out, overwhelmed and seething in resentment. It is hardly beneficial for you or the people you love, and you are also modelling behaviour that will make them vulnerable to their own depletion and compromised self-worth.

Rather than aiming for selflessness, let's get granular about what we're aspiring to. When we're trying to be selfless, what we're really trying to do is to be present, available, compassionate, understanding, caring, nurturing, loving, kind, and patient, right? Please ask yourself, what do you need to be this version of yourself? Most humans need decent sleep, good hydration and nutrition, relaxation, movement, time in nature, social connection, and we even need PLEASURE to resource us. Can you see how our phobia of being seen as selfish, our reverence of selflessness, keeps us stuck in a shame spiral where we can never truly meet the needs of those around us if haven't also had our needs met? Your denial serves no one. Your replenishment serves everyone!

And if the feeling of not being enough, of being undeserving, stops you in your tracks, please know that the feeling of worth comes *from* the nourishing action. So please, make time for your ease, make space for your relaxation. Allow yourself to say 'no' so that you can prioritize your sleep or your *joy*. Your boundaries with self and others are fundamental to you showing up as you aspire to, and rather than robbing others of your generosity, will facilitate you being more present and alive in your relationships. It is a genuine win–win.

How to feel confident to say no:

- Make the distinction between your capability and your capacity and know that you are your most precious resource.
- Remember, it's not unkind to have limits.
- In saying 'yes' to this thing, what are you saying 'no' to, and what long-term impact might this have?
- You don't need to over-explain and you also don't need approval or endorsement to honour yourself.
- Forgive yourself, darling, and then forgive yourself again. Sometimes the hardest disappointment to sit with is your own, and remember, disappointment doesn't mean you are doing something wrong.
- Tenderly place a hand on your heart to soothe yourself. You are safe. The fact that you care so much proves that you are a good human. Perhaps we can take the pressure down here and just allow ourselves to be human.

I hope you have enjoyed reading the first half of this book and that you feel like you have been handed the tools to start optimizing your post-menopausal health and to help reduce the risk of a life burdened with chronic disease. I also hope that things don't feel overly complicated or overwhelming. Much of this book is about getting back to basics, and the shifts outlined in each chapter are very similar. Try and follow your intuition and not be tempted to spend a fortune on unnecessary wellness 'kit' because real food, friendship, nature, meditation, breathwork, saunas and cold-water dipping don't cost the earth, and some of them cost nothing at all (although a weeklong trip to a Swiss wellness retreat would be lovely!). The Longevity Journal on the following pages is there to help you reflect on where you are and how you are going to start taking better care of yourself. What will you let go of, to create space for something new to grow?

Please go gently with yourself and trust your inner intelligence. The longevity world is so very male, and I hope this has given you a softer, more female approach, where eating real food, community, connection, purpose and nature matters the most.

the longevity journal

to document the journey with kindness and growing wisdom

HOW AM I GOING TO TAKE CARE OF MYSELF TODAY?

HOW AM I GOING TO BRING AWARENESS
TO MY SELF-NOURISHMENT?

HOW AM I GOING TO SET BOUNDARIES, SO I DON'T BURN OUT?

HOW AM I GOING TO FEED MYSELF TODAY?

HOW DO I FEEL AFTER A NOURISHING MEAL?

WHAT AM I GOING TO LET GO OF?

WHAT DO I WANT IN THIS SPACE I HAVE CREATED?

WHAT DID 'EATING WELL' MEAN TO ME BEFORE AND WHAT DOES IT MEAN NOW?

WHAT MAKES ME MORE CONNECTED TO MYSELF?

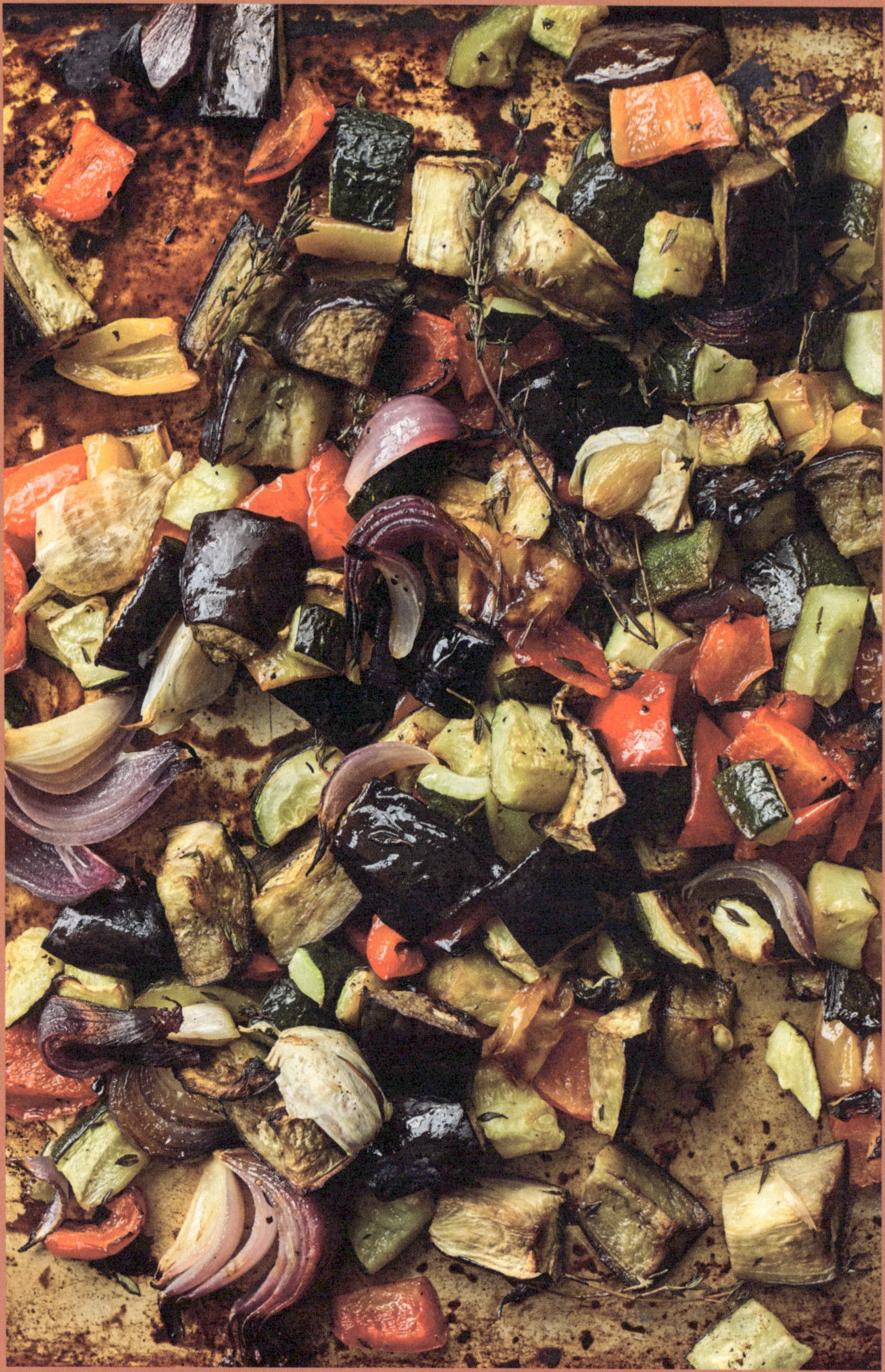

THE RECIPES

baked oats with spiced blackberries

avocado and kale pesto on toast with poached eggs

okinawan-style miso soup

fennel and flageolet salad

pearl barley and brothy bean soup with kale and almond pesto

roasted ginger and coconut tomatoes with white beans and sea bass

herbaceous kraut by rachel de thample

shakshuka-style lamb and aubergine with herbaceous kraut

metabolic harmony

LONGEVITY 7 LARDER

SERVES 1

Oats get a glow-up! Fibre-rich oats are combined with additional protein sources – the egg, yogurt, pumpkin seeds and walnuts – and coupled with antioxidants from the spices and the blackberries. This will keep cravings at bay all morning.

baked oats with spiced blackberries

Butter or neutral oil, for greasing
40g/1½oz rolled oats
1 egg, lightly beaten
½ tsp ground cinnamon
½ tsp ground cardamom
⅓ tsp baking powder
1 tsp maple syrup
1 tbsp pumpkin seeds
1 tbsp walnut pieces
50g/1¾oz frozen blackberries (frozen cherries or blueberries also work well)
50ml/2fl oz milk of your choice

TO SERVE
2–3 tbsp natural yogurt of your choice
1 tsp maple syrup, to drizzle

1. Preheat the oven to 180°C fan/400°F/Gas 6. Grease a 240ml/8½fl oz (10cm/4in diameter) ramekin with butter or oil.

2. Mix all the remaining ingredients together in a bowl, then pour into the greased ramekin.

3. Bake for 20–25 minutes until risen. Serve with the yogurt and the drizzle of maple syrup to the side.

COOK'S NOTES

Swap the pumpkin seeds for hemp seeds or sunflower seeds.

You can use crushed hazelnuts or almond slivers instead of the walnut pieces, if you like.

LONGEVITY 9 LARDER

SERVES 2

This recipe provides a simple way to up your polyphenols at breakfast time, with the pesto containing beta carotene in the kale and oleuropein and hydroxytyrosol in the olive oil. The pesto provides plentiful vitamins and minerals, too, including vitamin K, calcium and magnesium, along with protein from the eggs and beneficial fats from the avocado and the olive oil.

avocado and kale pesto on toast with poached eggs

- 2 eggs
- 1 slice of your favourite bread
- 1 small or ½ medium ripe avocado, peeled and stoned
- 2 tbsp Kale and Almond Pesto (see p.135)
- Butter, softened, for spreading
- Black pepper

1. Poach your eggs to your liking, either in a pan of simmering water or using an egg poacher or poacher cups. Toast your bread.

2. While your eggs are poaching and your bread is toasting, mash the avocado in a small bowl and swirl in the pesto.

3. Butter your toast, spoon over the avocado and pesto mix, top with your poached eggs and finish with a good crack of black pepper.

COOK'S NOTE

Serve soft-boiled eggs (peeled and halved) in place of the poached eggs, if you prefer. Cook them in simmering water for 6½ minutes for the perfect jammy eggs.

LONGEVITY 9 LARDER

SERVES 2

This dish usually uses a purple sweet potato known as *beni imo*, which is used a lot in Okinawan cookery. The easier to find orange variety makes a good substitute. Both are great sources of fibre and purple sweet potatoes are rich in anthocyanins that you find in blueberries; the orange variety are high in the antioxidant beta carotene. The miso is added right at the end so that the heat of the cooking doesn't kill off its beneficial bacteria. Perfect as a simple lunch or a light supper.

okinawan-style miso soup

DASHI BROTH

1 litre/1¾ pints water
1 large strip of dried kombu
6 dried shiitake mushrooms

MISO SOUP

8g fresh ginger, peeled and thinly sliced into matchsticks
½ medium sweet potato, peeled and cut into 1.5cm/⅝in cubes
40g/1½oz frozen edamame beans
10g dried daikon radish
2 spring onions, separated into white and green parts, finely sliced
1 x 300g/10½oz packet silken or medium-firm tofu, drained and cut into 1.5cm/⅝in cubes
2 tbsp white miso paste

1. Put all the dashi broth ingredients into a pan and bring to the boil. Reduce the heat, partially cover the pan and simmer for 30 minutes, or for up to an hour for a stronger taste.

2. After 30 or 60 minutes, add the ginger and sweet potato cubes to the broth. If you prefer sliced shiitake, remove them from the pan, cool and slice, then return them to the broth. Simmer with the pan partially covered, and after 4 minutes, add the edamame beans, radish and the white parts of the spring onions and simmer for 6 minutes.

3. Carefully add the tofu cubes so they don't break up. Allow them to warm through for 1–2 minutes. Check that the sweet potato is cooked – it should be tender but not falling apart.

4. Turn off the heat. Take a ladleful of the broth and pour it into a small bowl, then add the miso. Whisk gently until dissolved and then add it back into the pan and gently mix in. Ladle the soup into two bowls, keeping the kombu in the pan, sprinkle over the green parts of the spring onions and serve.

COOK'S NOTES

The dashi broth can be replaced with bone broth or vegetable stock, if you're pushed for time – simply heat through before adding the ginger and sweet potato.

LONGEVITY 11 LARDER

SERVES 4

A kind of beany Caesar salad, filled with plant protein and fibre. The dill provides the polyphenols quercetin and kaempferol, along with vitamin C, the walnuts are a rich source of vitamin E and the polyphenol ellagic acid and catechins (also found in green tea), the rocket is a rich source of quercetin, beta carotene and vitamin C, and the beans are a brilliant source of potassium and fibre.

fennel and flageolet salad

- 1 large courgette, thinly sliced
- 1 large fennel bulb, trimmed and thinly sliced
- 1 tbsp olive oil
- 1 tbsp lemon juice
- 10g/¼oz fresh dill, roughly chopped
- 1 x 400g/14oz can flageolet beans, drained (but keep hold of the liquid for the dressing) and rinsed
- 40g/1½oz rocket or lamb's lettuce
- 35g/1¼oz Pecorino or Parmesan cheese, thinly shaved
- 40g/1½oz walnuts, toasted (see Cook's Note on p.182) and roughly chopped
- Salt and black pepper

DRESSING

- 3 tbsp aquafaba (the drained liquid from the can of flageolet beans)
- 1½ tsp white wine vinegar or lemon juice
- 1 small garlic clove, crushed
- ½ tsp Dijon mustard
- 100ml/3½fl oz olive oil
- 15g/½oz canned anchovy fillets in oil (5–7 fillets, depending on size), drained and roughly chopped
- 50g/1¾oz Pecorino or Parmesan cheese, finely grated
- Black pepper

1. Add the courgette and fennel to a large bowl with the olive oil, lemon juice, ½ teaspoon of salt and a good grind of black pepper. Mix well to combine – use your hands to massage in the oil and lemon – and then set aside for about 20 minutes to soften.

2. Meanwhile, make the dressing. Place the aquafaba, vinegar or lemon juice, garlic and Dijon mustard in the small bowl of a food processor. With the machine on, slowly pour in the olive oil, until thick. Add the anchovies, cheese and the black pepper and blitz just a couple of times, to combine.

3. When ready to serve, add half of the dressing (keep the rest – see Cook's Notes on p.132) to the bowl with the courgette and fennel, along with the dill and beans. Mix well and then add the rocket or lamb's lettuce, shaved cheese and toasted walnuts. Give everything one more gentle mix, transfer to a big platter and serve.

recipe continues overleaf

COOK'S NOTES

You can add a cooked fillet of trout or salmon or a jar of tuna, or to continue with the Caesar salad vibe, add in some grilled chicken, if you like.

A mandoline is your friend here for slicing the courgette and fennel as thin as they love to be, but do be careful! To shave the cheese thinly, use a vegetable peeler.

All sorts of nuts work as well as the walnuts here – pine nuts and pistachios are both great.

You'll make twice as much dressing as you need for this salad. Keep the rest in an airtight jar or bowl in the refrigerator for up to 3 days, ready for the next salad. Chicken, trout and hard-boiled eggs all love this dressing.

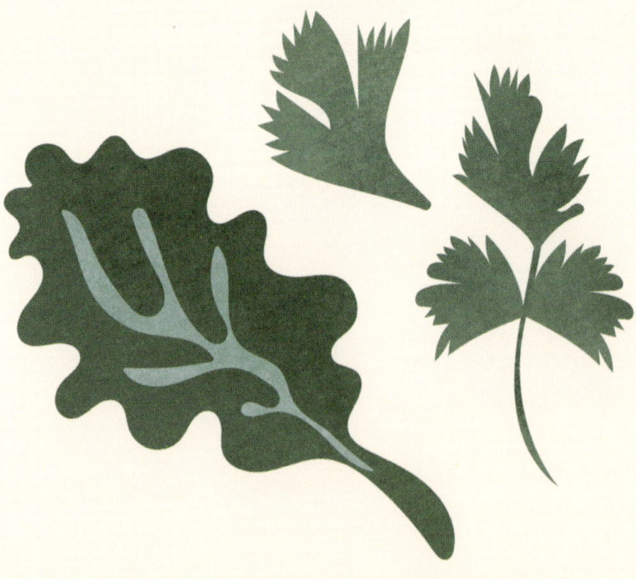

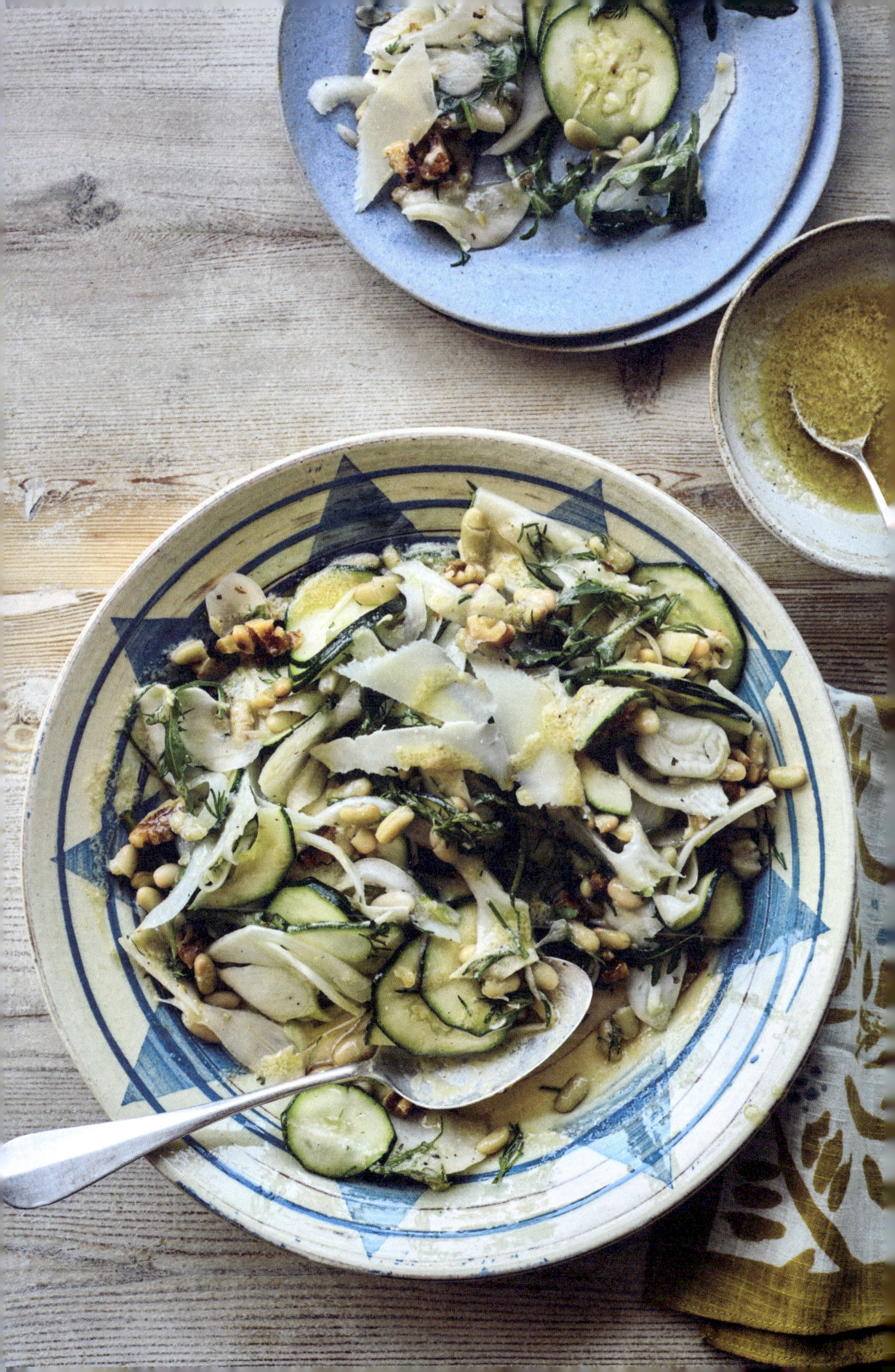

LONGEVITY 18 LARDER

SERVES 4*

(*with leftover pesto)

I went to Scotland for the first time recently and I was not only blown away by the Highlands but also the traditional food culture, including simple Scotch broth kits that you could buy in every supermarket – nutrient-rich, simple to make and cheap. My take is high in fibre, and contains antioxidants including beta carotene and quercetin. The pesto contains antibacterial allicin, from the garlic; iron, vitamin K, calcium and magnesium from the kale; and vitamin E from the almonds.

pearl barley and brothy bean soup with kale and almond pesto

- 4 tbsp olive oil, plus extra for drizzling to serve
- 1 large onion, cut into 1.5cm/⅝in dice
- 1 medium fennel bulb, trimmed and cut into 1.5cm/⅝in dice
- 1 large carrot, peeled and cut into 1.5cm/⅝in dice
- 3 celery sticks, cut into 1.5cm/⅝in dice
- 2 garlic cloves, crushed
- 1 tbsp fresh thyme leaves, chopped
- 1 tbsp tomato purée
- 1 tsp ground allspice
- 1½ tsp ground cumin
- 1.2–1.5 litres/2–2¾ pints vegetable stock
- 1 x 400g/14oz can chopped tomatoes
- 100g/3½oz pearl barley, rinsed
- 2 bay leaves
- 1 x 400g/14oz can white beans (cannellini, chickpeas or butter beans), drained and rinsed
- Salt and black pepper

1. Add the olive oil to a large saucepan and place over a medium heat. Add the onion, fennel, carrot and celery and cook for about 8 minutes, stirring a few times, for the vegetables to soften. Add the garlic, thyme, tomato purée and ground spices, along with a pinch of salt and a good grind of black pepper. Cook for another 4 minutes, stirring every now and then, adding a little of the stock (or white wine, if there is a bottle open) if things are starting to catch in the pan.

2. Add the canned tomatoes, pearl barley, bay leaves and the remaining stock and bring to the boil. Reduce to a simmer and then cook gently, partially covered, for about 40 minutes, until the pearl barley is cooked through and the vegetables are nice and soft.

3. Meanwhile, make the pesto. Add the kale, parsley, oregano, almonds and garlic to a food processor and pulse until finely chopped. Add the olive oil, along with the salt and black pepper and pulse to a coarse paste. Transfer to a clean sealed jar and keep in the refrigerator until ready to use.

4. Add the canned beans to the soup and cook for a final 5 minutes, then discard the bay leaves. Serve the soup in bowls, with a generous spoonful of pesto swirled through each portion and a final drizzle of olive oil.

KALE AND ALMOND PESTO

50g/1¾oz curly kale leaves, roughly chopped
30g/1oz fresh parsley leaves
10g/¼oz fresh oregano leaves
50g/1¾oz blanched almonds, lightly toasted
2 small garlic cloves, roughly chopped
4 tbsp olive oil
½ tsp salt
Black pepper

COOK'S NOTES

This soup is a mix of a Scotch broth and a Tuscan ribollita, the literal translation of which is 're-boiled' – so treat it as a bit of a refrigerator raid. Use what veg you have hanging around – parsnip instead of carrot, leek instead of fennel, for example. It's worth taking time to dice the veg nice and small and even – 1.5cm/⅝in dice work well – so that the soup cooks evenly and looks good.

If you want to make this gluten-free, then buckwheat groats would work instead of the pearl barley, as would adding some cooked quinoa (I like the pre-cooked packets for ease, and add them with the canned beans towards the end). Use gluten-free veg stock, too.

You'll make more pesto than you need, but it keeps well in the refrigerator for 3–4 days. Store it in the jar, drizzle over a thin layer of olive oil and close the lid. Use it for the Avocado and Kale Pesto on Toast with Poached Eggs (see p.129) and the Posh Baked Beans with Feta and Kale and Almond Pesto (see p.200).

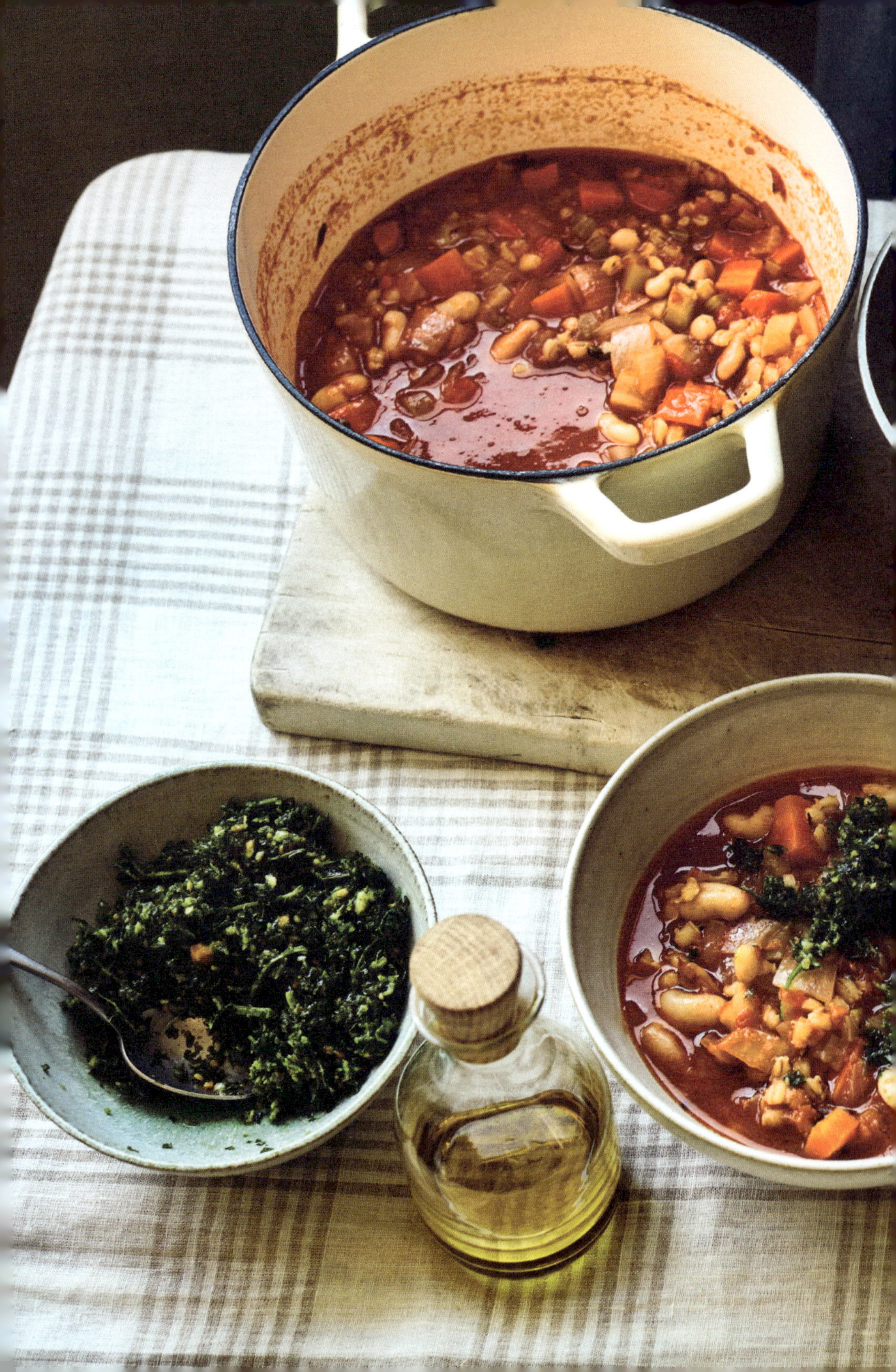

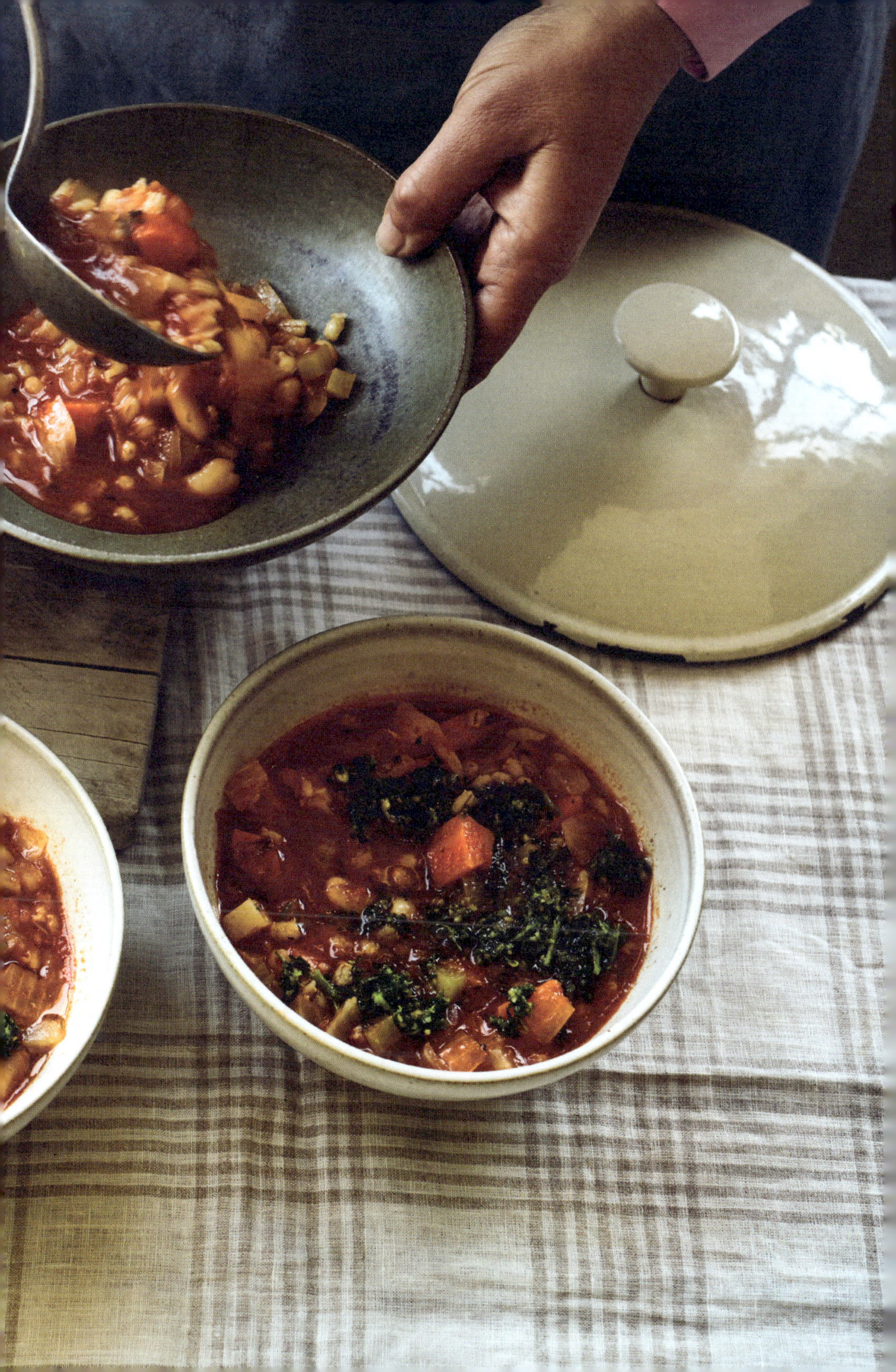

LONGEVITY 9 LARDER

SERVES 4

This simple one-pot dish is warming and super-nourishing. The cherry tomatoes are a great source of the antioxidant lycopene, the ginger is a natural anti-inflammatory and antioxidant, the coriander provides vitamins A, C and K, and the butter beans provide plant-based protein and fibre. You can also top the fish with the Coriander–Walnut Pesto used in the Red Lentil and Harissa Soup recipe on p.172.

roasted ginger and coconut tomatoes with white beans and sea bass

1kg/2lb 4oz cherry tomatoes
250ml/9fl oz coconut milk
30g/1oz fresh ginger, peeled and coarsely grated
30g/1oz fresh coriander, leaves and stalks roughly chopped
2 tsp Aleppo chilli flakes (or 1 tsp regular chilli flakes)
4 garlic cloves, peeled and left whole
1 tbsp maple syrup (or runny honey)
1½ tsp ground turmeric
1 x 400g/14oz can butter beans (or chickpeas or white beans), rinsed and drained
sea bass (or cod or halibut) fillets (about 360g/12½oz total weight), skin on
Salt and black pepper

TO SERVE

1 lemon or lime, quartered
Coconut yogurt (optional)
5g/⅛oz fresh coriander leaves

1. Preheat the oven to 230°C fan/480°F/Gas 9 (or as close to this as your oven will go).

2. Place the first eight ingredients in an ovenproof baking dish (about 30 x 20cm/12 x 8in), along with a pinch of salt and a good grind of black pepper and mix well. Roast for 30 minutes, stirring halfway through, until the tomatoes are charred.

3. Stir in the butter beans and then lay the fish fillets on top, skin-side down. Spoon some of the sauce over the top of the fish and then return to the oven for a final 10 minutes.

4. Serve directly from the dish, with the wedges of lemon or lime alongside, along with a spoonful of coconut yogurt (if using) and the coriander leaves sprinkled on top.

COOK'S NOTES

The tomato and bean mixture is also great by itself (without the fish) – as a side to all sorts of eggs or piled on toast with slices of avocado. Serve it with plain rice, or with crusty bread to mop up the juices, and a big green salad.

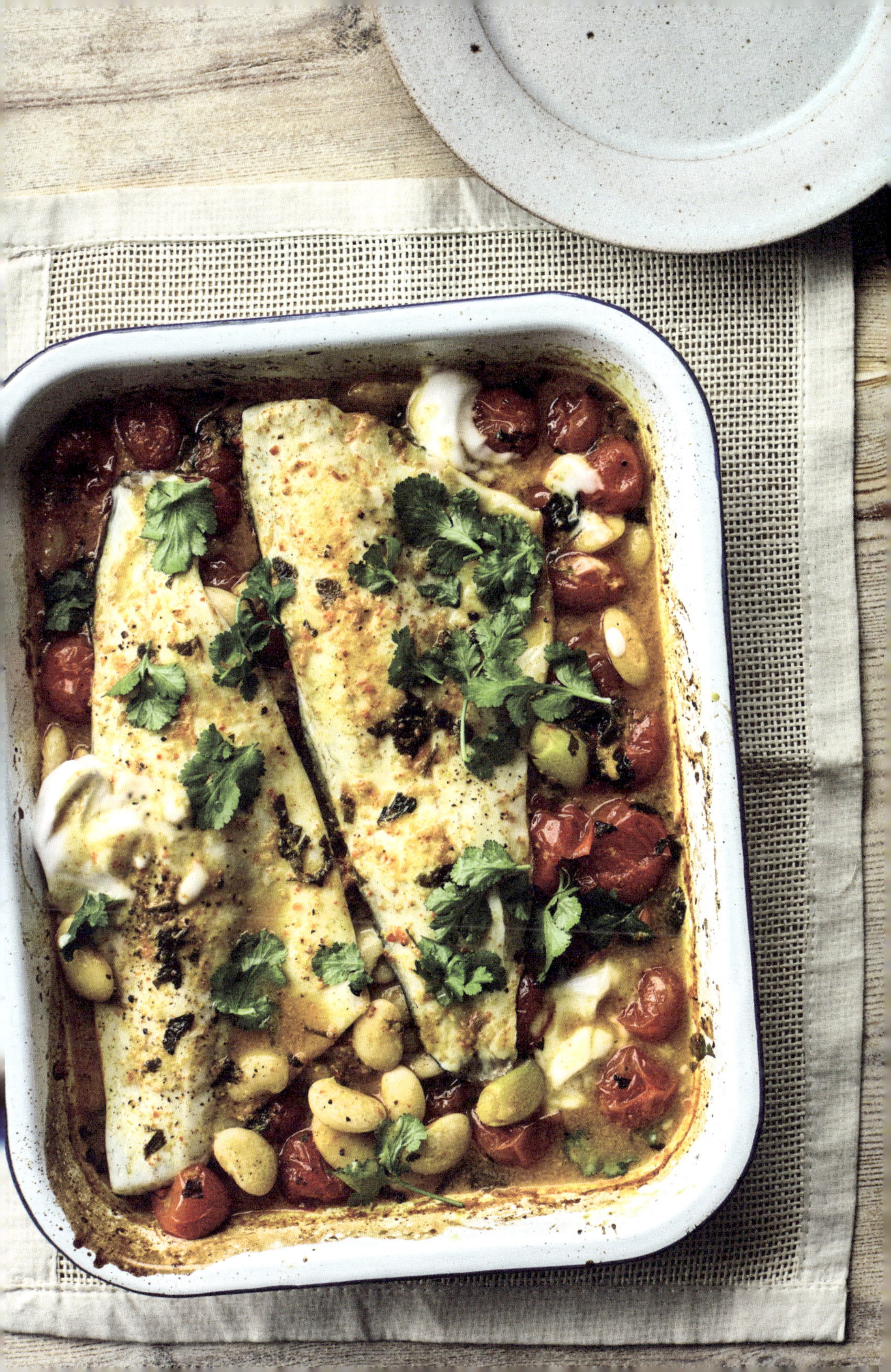

LONGEVITY & LARDER

MAKES 500g*

(*1lb 2oz)

Sauerkraut's magic is that it is wonderful simple yet wild complex both at the same time. In essence, it's just two ingredients: cabbage and salt. The former shredded with the latter massaged into its cell walls to draw out the moisture, softening it enough to fold into a jar, nicely compact and then the magic happens. The natural bacteria on the cabbage start to break down the brassica's sugars and fibres, making it easier for us to digest, as well as helping us assimilate the incredible nutritional diversity found in the cabbage.

It's rich in vitamin C and when you ferment it, you get up to 50 per cent more of this immune-boosting nutrient than if you were to just eat it raw. Adding herbs to the mix not only offers a beautifully aromatic, palate-pleasing boost, it also enriches sauerkraut's healing powers. Use any of the herbs listed, all revered for their role in healthy Mediterranean diets, or just choose your favourite one.

The herbal addition leans in more to summery Italian and Greek territory and I love pairing this kraut with either cold or warm freshly cooked chickpeas, cannellini beans or gigantes. Finished with a peppery olive oil, it's a wildly delicious dish on its own or paired with grilled fish or lamb.

herbaceous kraut

by Rachel de Thample

Fermenter, forager and author

- 500g/1lb 2oz cabbage (such as spring pointed cabbage, white or green cabbage, or you can use red cabbage here, too)
- 10g/¼oz salt, plus 4g/⅛oz extra for the brine
- Large handful of fresh herbs (10–15g/¼–½oz leaves only, without stalks), such as oregano, thyme, rosemary, basil, fennel (fronds and/or seeds) and/or mint
- 7–8 bay leaves

1. Strip one or two larger outer leaves from your cabbage and reserve. Thinly shred the rest of your cabbage. Pile it into a large bowl with the 10g/¼oz of salt. Strip the oregano, thyme and/or rosemary from their stalks (if using these). Roughly chop the rosemary; the oregano and thyme leaves can go in whole. Add them to the bowl. If using basil, fennel and/or mint, roughly chop or tear them before adding to the mix. Add the bay leaves whole.

2. Then, get your hands stuck in there and massage and scrunch the salt into the herby cabbage – it's incredible aromatherapy. Once the cabbage is juicy and softened, about 5 minutes, pack it into a clean jam jar with a twist-off lid (see Cook's Note), adding the kraut little by little, packing down each layer as you go. The key is to ensure you keep as much air out as possible.

3. Use the reserved cabbage leaves to cover the compacted cabbage. Press down til there's a good layer of liquid and top with extra brine (made by mixing 100ml/3½fl oz of cold water with the extra 4g/⅛oz of salt) until the brine comes right to the top of the jar, then secure with a lid.

4. Keep in a dry spot at room temperature for 2 weeks. Check daily to ensure the brining liquid is always covering the cabbage and that none of the cabbage is exposed to air.

5. After 2 weeks, it's ready to eat straight away or you can leave it at room temperature to ferment further, or pop it in the refrigerator until you're ready to eat it. So long as it's fully covered in the brining liquid it'll keep for months in the refrigerator.

COOK'S NOTE

Burping the jar during fermentation (to release the build-up of gases) is only necessary if using a Kilner jar with a clip lid and rubber ring, so my recommended jar would be a normal jam jar with a twist-off lid – the building gases can happily escape these jars/lids without the need to burp. Burping is only necessary if the jar is hissing, which just means a little twist of the lid will help release building gases, then you can refasten the lid.

LONGEVITY
17
LARDER

SERVES
4

Some of the longest-living people on the planet adhere to a mainly plant-based diet, but they do eat meat occasionally, and if they do it's never the main part of a dish. Like this shakshuka made with lamb mince and bursting with longevity-loving vegetables, spices, herbs and tahini. Serve it with either Rachel de Thample's beautiful Herbaceous Kraut (see p.140), or try the shop-bought version given here.

shakshuka-style lamb and aubergine with herbaceous kraut

2 aubergines
2 tbsp olive oil
1 onion, finely chopped
4 garlic cloves, crushed
2 tbsp tomato purée
2 tsp ground cumin
1 tsp ground allspice
½ tsp ground cinnamon
1 tsp Aleppo chilli flakes (or ½ tsp regular chilli flakes), plus extra to serve
200g/7oz canned chopped tomatoes
400g/14oz fresh lamb mince
4 spring onions, white parts only, chopped
30g/1oz fresh coriander leaves, roughly chopped
20g/¾oz fresh mint leaves, shredded
4 eggs
Salt and black pepper

1. To chargrill the aubergines, either put them directly over a gas flame or in a chargrill pan. Directly over a flame they will take 18–20 minutes, turning with tongs throughout to get charred on all sides. In a preheated hot chargrill pan over a high heat they'll take 35–40 minutes, turning occasionally throughout (it's also worth ventilating the kitchen while you are chargrilling – open a window or an outside door or turn on ventilation). Either way, once done, transfer the charred aubergines to a colander set over a bowl, make a vertical slit down one side of each of them and leave to cool and drain.

2. Once cool, scoop out the flesh – there should be about 290g/10oz in total – and keep this in the colander to continue to drain. The skin can be discarded.

3. Place all the ingredients for the herby sauerkraut (if using) in a bowl and mix to combine. Set aside.

4. Place all the ingredients for the tahini sauce (if using) in a small bowl and mix to combine. Set aside.

HERBY SAUERKRAUT (SHOP-BOUGHT VERSION), OR USE THE HERBACEOUS KRAUT RECIPE (SEE P.140)

- 150g/5½oz shop-bought sauerkraut
- 15g/½oz fresh mint leaves, shredded
- 10g/¼oz fresh dill, finely chopped
- 10g/¼oz fresh coriander, finely chopped

TAHINI SAUCE (OPTIONAL)

- 80g/3oz tahini
- 70ml/2½fl oz water
- 1 tbsp lemon juice
- 1 garlic clove, crushed
- ¼ tsp ground cumin
- ½ tsp salt

5. Heat the olive oil in a medium sauté pan over a medium-high heat. Add the onion and cook for 4 minutes, stirring a few times. Add the garlic, tomato purée, ground spices, chilli flakes, ½ teaspoon of salt and a good grind of black pepper. Cook for another 4 minutes and then add the chopped tomatoes and lamb mince. Cook for another 5 minutes, stirring constantly to break down the meat, then add the aubergine flesh, spring onions and herbs and stir through to wilt.

6. Make four wells in the mixture. Crack an egg into each well, cover the pan and cook over a medium heat for 8 minutes, until the egg whites are set but the yolks are still runny.

7. Serve straight from the pan, with a big spoonful of herby sauerkraut alongside and a drizzle of tahini sauce on top (if using).

COOK'S NOTES

The shakshuka mixture can be taken up to the point just before the eggs are added and can be made a day or two ahead, for a supper that's then ready in less than 15 minutes. Simply cool, store in an airtight container or the covered pan in the refrigerator, then reheat gently until piping hot before cracking in the eggs and finishing as above. The herby sauerkraut (if making your own) and tahini sauce are best made fresh on the day of serving.

Other fresh minced meat can be used instead of the lamb – fresh chicken thigh mince works really well, for example.

The tahini sauce is lovely but the dish still tastes wonderful without it!

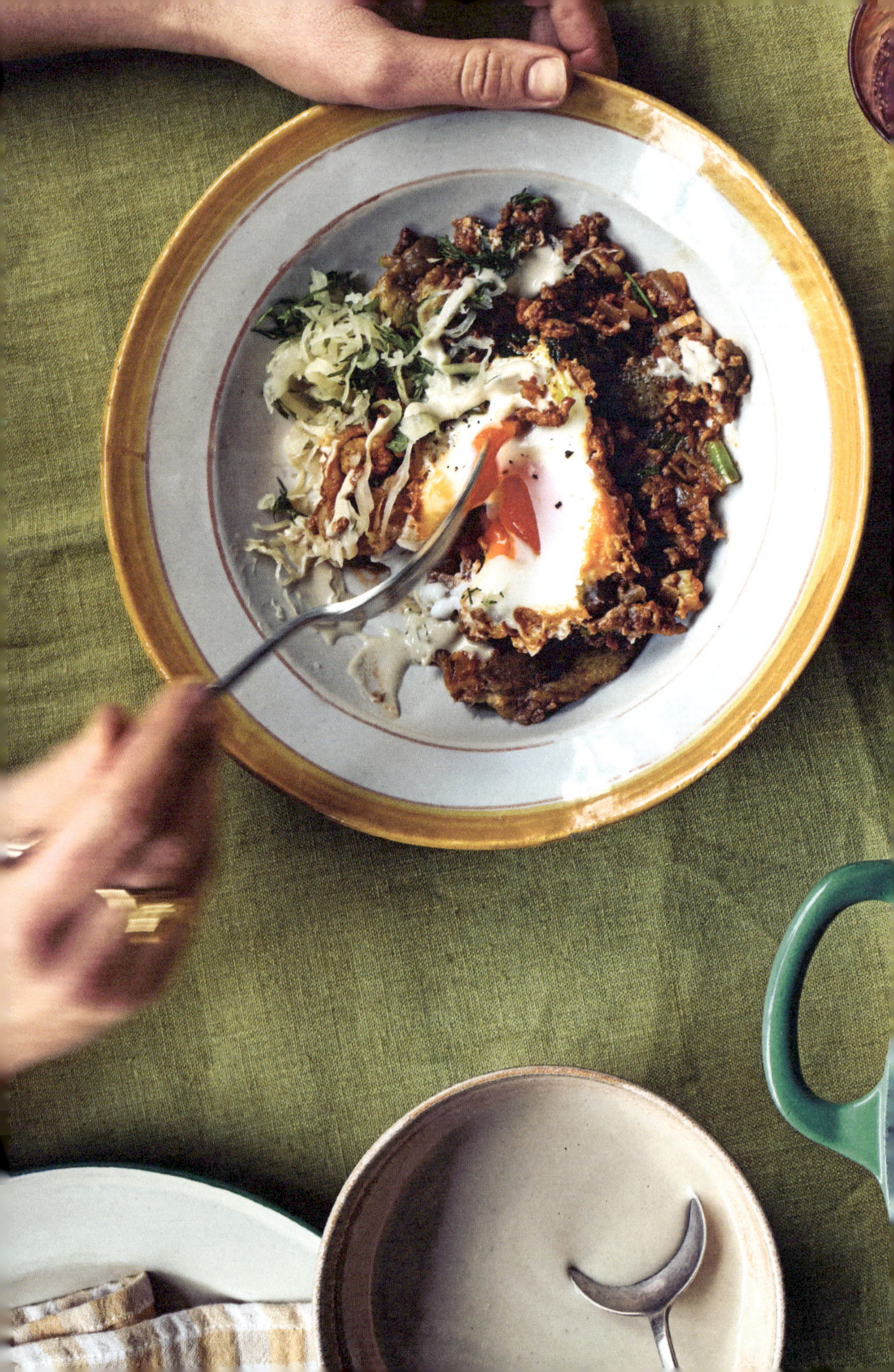

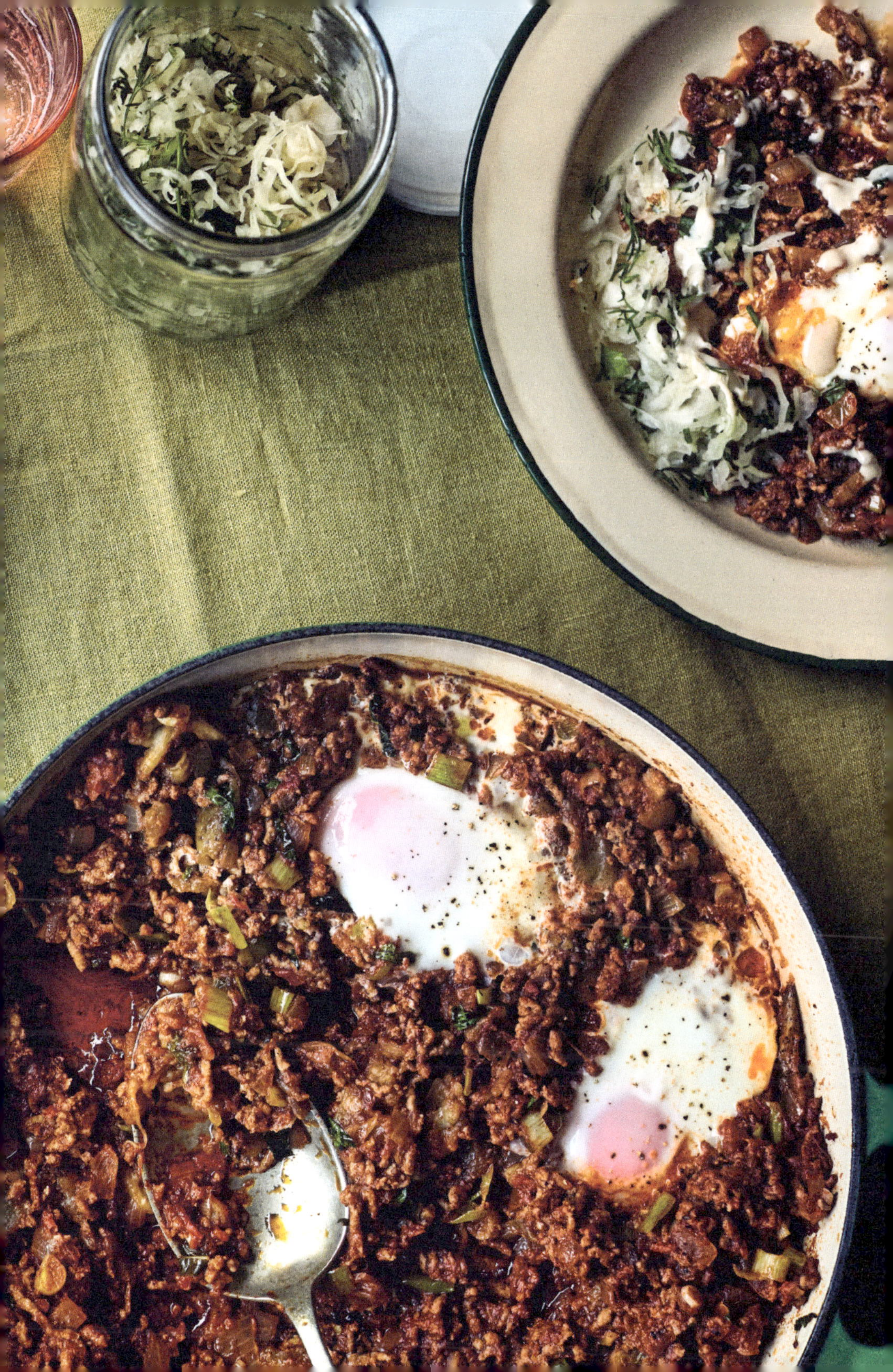

under pressure

queen
of hearts

LONGEVITY 6 LARDER

SERVES 1

Delivering nitric oxide from the beetroot, antioxidant vitamin C from the orange and pomegranate, antioxidant beta carotene from the carrots, gingerols from the ginger, and curcumin from the fresh turmeric., this juice packs a punch with ingredients that help support blood pressure and keep our blood vessels healthy.

under pressure

2 fresh beetroots
2 medium carrots
30g/1oz fresh ginger
15g/½oz fresh turmeric
1 orange, peeled and roughly chopped
1 pomegranate, seeds extracted

1. There is no need to peel the beetroots, carrots, ginger and turmeric. Simply wash them, then chop them to fit into your juicer. Add the orange and pomegranate seeds, and juice.

2. Pour into a glass and enjoy.

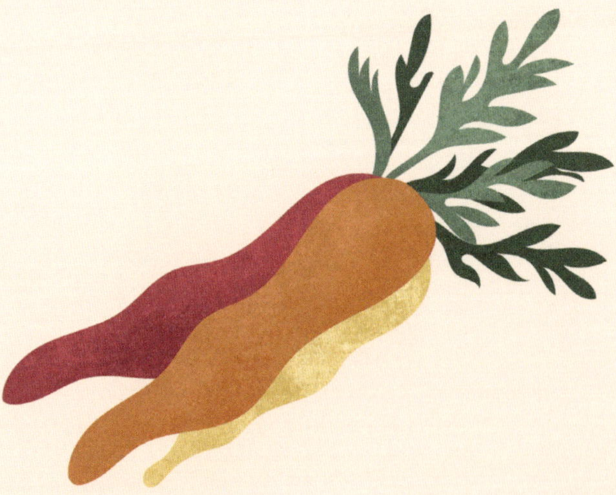

LONGEVITY 8 LARDER

SERVES 1

An antioxidant-packed breakfast! The blackberries contain anthocyanins, responsible for the dark purple/black pigment. The almond butter is a great source of antioxidant vitamin E, while the cacao provides flavanols such as catechins and procyanidins. Chia seeds and Greek-style yogurt provide protein, to help keep low blood sugar at bay, which can stimulate vasoconstriction and higher blood pressure.

blackberry, acai and cacao chia pot

50g/1¾oz frozen blackberries
½–1 tsp maple syrup (depending on how sweet you like things)
½ tsp acai powder
2 tsp cacao powder
150ml/5fl oz milk of your choice
2 tbsp chia seeds
3–4 tbsp Greek-style yogurt or plant-based alternative (soy works well)
2 tsp almond butter

TO SERVE
1 tsp ground linseed/flaxseed
1 tsp pumpkin seeds

1. Blend the frozen blackberries, maple syrup, acai and cacao powders, and milk together in a blender. Tip the mixture into a medium bowl (that you can fit in your refrigerator), add the chia seeds and stir well. Cover the bowl and leave the seeds to soak in the refrigerator overnight (or for at least 20 minutes, if you are short of time).

2. Remove the bowl from the refrigerator and stir well. Spoon half the mixture into a clean jar, followed by half the yogurt and 1 teaspoon of the almond butter, then repeat the layers.

3. Top the jar with the ground linseed/flaxseed and pumpkin seeds, and serve.

COOK'S NOTES

You can switch the frozen blackberries for frozen raspberries or blueberries, if you like.

Chopped almonds work well instead of the pumpkin seeds to serve.

LONGEVITY 6 LARDER

MAKES 12

A nod to my fave from the British chain Gail's Bakery, combining antioxidant-rich cacao with delicious and highly nutritious tahini. These are gluten-free and close to being sugar-free, too, and if you use soy or oat milk they are vegan as well. You make a 'flax egg' by mixing ground linseed/flaxseed with water, which approximates the addition of an egg when baking. After a few minutes, its consistency turns 'gloopy' and this acts as a binder when mixed with other ingredients.

cacao tahini bites

20g/¾oz ground linseed/flaxseed
2 tbsp warm water
80g/3oz ground almonds
¾ tsp baking powder
½ tsp bicarbonate of soda
25g/1oz cacao powder
¼ tsp salt
200ml/7fl oz full-fat milk (soy milk, if vegan)
80g/3oz dark chocolate (70 per cent cocoa solids), broken up into small pieces
60g/2¼oz tahini
50g/1¾oz ripe banana flesh (½ small banana), mashed until smooth
½ tsp vanilla bean paste or extract
1 tbsp maple syrup
1 tbsp sesame seeds (a mix of black and white looks great, or else just white)

1. Preheat the oven to 180°C fan/400°F/Gas 6. Line a cupcake tin with 12 paper cases.

2. Mix together the ground linseed/flaxseed with the warm water in a small bowl and set aside until needed.

3. Sift together the ground almonds, baking powder, bicarbonate of soda, cacao powder and salt into a large bowl and set aside.

4. Warm the milk in a small saucepan over a medium heat until bubbles appear. Pour the warm milk over the chocolate in a separate heatproof bowl, leave for a minute and then stir to combine. Once it's smooth, stir in the tahini, banana, vanilla, maple syrup and the linseed/flaxseed–water mix and then add to the bowl with the dry ingredients. Fold together just to combine.

5. Divide the mixture between the cupcake cases. Sprinkle the sesame seeds over the tops.

6. Bake for 12 minutes (or 10 minutes, if making cookies, see Cook's Notes, see overleaf), or until the tops are just set. Remove from the oven and leave to cool completely in the cupcake tin before serving.

recipe continues overleaf

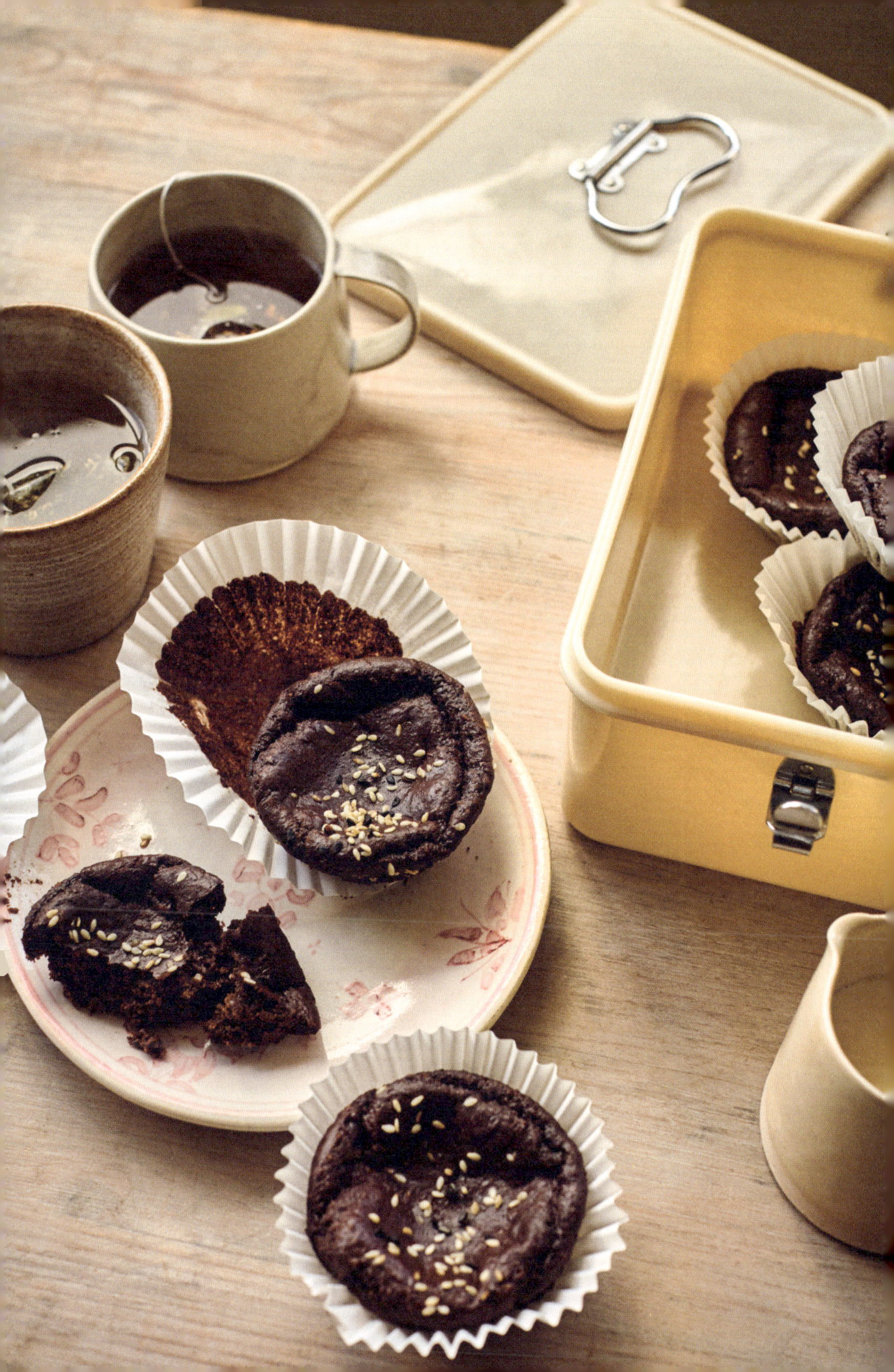

COOK'S NOTES

These can either be made into little cupcakes or you can spoon the mixture directly onto a baking paper-lined baking tray to make 12 cookies. These need to be baked for 10 minutes.

These bites will keep in an airtight container at room temperature for 3–4 days (1–2 days if made with ground hazelnuts – see below).

You can use ground hazelnuts in place of the ground almonds, but these bites will dry out more quickly, so are best eaten within a day or two.

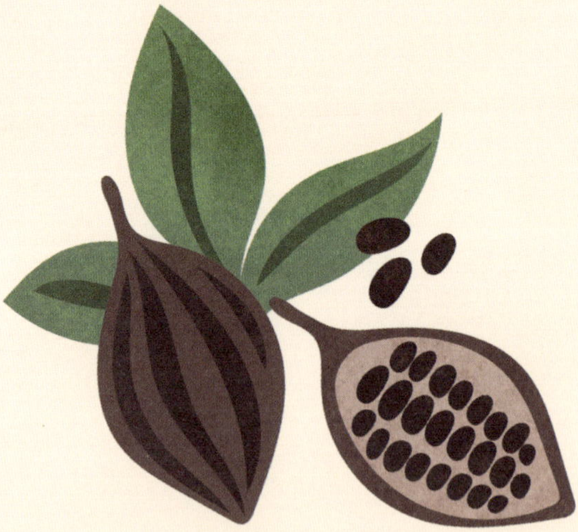

LONGEVITY 13 LARDER

SERVES 2

I eat this when I am starting to feel a cold coming on – you can add more ginger and turmeric if you want to give yourself some extra heat to blast away the lurgy! Both ginger and turmeric are potent anti-inflammatories, and the tofu adds a little plant protein to help support your immune system even further.

turmeric, tofu and ginger noodle soup

1 tsp coriander seeds
4 black peppercorns
1 onion, peeled and halved
25g/1oz fresh ginger, finely sliced (no need to peel)
10g/¼oz fresh turmeric, sliced (no need to peel), or ½ tsp ground turmeric
3 garlic cloves, peeled and roughly crushed with the side of a knife
2 small carrots, halved (no need to peel)
750ml/1¼ pints hot vegetable or chicken stock
200g/7oz dried noodles of your choice – I like to use flat rice noodles
300g/10½oz silken tofu, drained and carefully cut into 2cm/¾in chunks
40g/1½oz mangetout

TO SERVE
2 spring onions, finely sliced
Juice of ½ lemon
Tamari

1. Add the coriander seeds, peppercorns, onion halves and sliced ginger and turmeric to a lidded saucepan (without the lid at this stage) over a medium heat and dry-fry for 2 minutes until lightly toasted and smelling fragrant. Add the garlic and carrots and continue to dry-fry for another 2 minutes before adding the hot vegetable or chicken stock.

2. Bring to the boil, then simmer for 25 minutes with the lid on. When it's ready, you should be able to smell all the glorious aromatics.

3. When the soup is almost ready to serve, cook the noodles according to the packet instructions, then drain and rinse them under cold water to stop them cooking further.

4. Divide the noodles into two bowls and add the tofu and mangetout on top. Strain the broth using a sieve as you ladle it over the noodles, to remove the aromatics (discard these). The mangetout will gently cook as you add the broth. Sprinkle over the spring onions, squeeze over the lemon juice, add a dash of tamari, and serve.

LONGEVITY 14 LARDER

SERVES 6*

(*as a dip or as part of a spread)

This is something I first tried in Istanbul. What a wonderful way to enjoy walnuts, rich in flavonoids and vitamin E as well as anti-inflammatory omega-3 oils. Walnuts are one of the earliest cultivated food sources on earth, thought to have been grown as early as 7000 BC. The Walnuts and Healthy Aging study – a randomized clinical trial carried out on elderly men and women with a history of hypertension from 2012 to 2014 – showed a change in systolic blood pressure when consuming walnuts daily.[113] Served with the Za'atar and Sesame Seed Crackers that follow, this is great on its own or as part of a spread.

muhammara

100g/3½oz walnuts
4 red peppers, quartered and deseeded
1 red onion, cut into 2cm/¾in-thick wedges
1 red chilli, halved lengthways and deseeded (optional)
1 tbsp roughly chopped fresh thyme leaves
4 large garlic cloves, skin on
3 tbsp olive oil
1½ tsp ground cumin
1 tbsp pomegranate molasses
2 tsp Aleppo chilli flakes (or 1 tsp regular chilli flakes)
2 tsp smoked paprika
1 tbsp lemon juice
Salt and black pepper
1 tbsp roughly chopped fresh parsley leaves, to serve

1. Preheat the oven to 160°C fan/350°F/Gas 4. Line two baking trays with baking paper.

2. Spread the walnuts out on one of the lined baking trays and roast for 8–10 minutes, until lightly toasted. Remove from the oven and, once cool, roughly chop, then reserve 20g/¾oz. Place the remaining 80g/3oz in a food processor and blitz until they form the texture of breadcrumbs.

3. Increase the oven temperature to 220°C fan/475°F/Gas 9. Add the peppers, onion, chilli (if using), thyme, garlic cloves and olive oil to the second lined baking tray, along with 1½ teaspoons of salt and a good grind of black pepper. Mix well and then roast for about 30 minutes, stirring halfway through, until the skin of the peppers is starting to blacken and the onion is soft and cooked through.

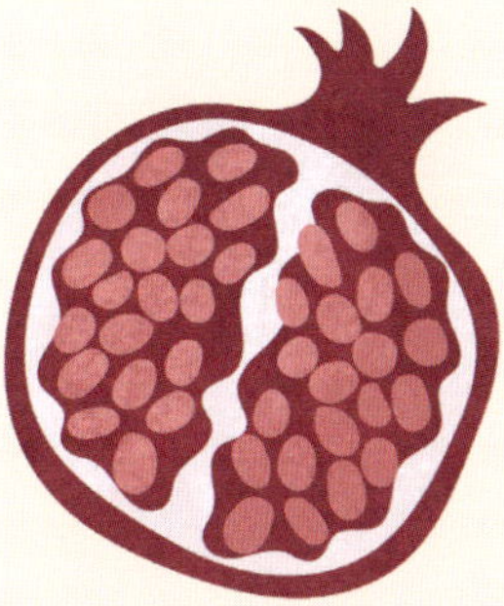

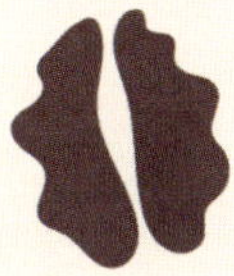

4. Remove from the oven. Squeeze the soft garlic cloves out of their skin and then transfer the roasted veg mix to a food processor (the skin can stay on the peppers as it adds texture), along with the blitzed nuts and all the remaining ingredients, except the parsley and reserved chopped nuts. Pulse a few times – you want to keep the texture coarse, so don't overdo it here.

5. Transfer the dip to a bowl or platter, sprinkle over the parsley and reserved chopped nuts and serve with the crackers (see overleaf).

COOK'S NOTES

This is lovely served as a dip as it is, but it can also be bulked out by either crumbling feta cheese or scooping thick Greek-style yogurt on top just before serving. Or try serving a layer of butter bean mash underneath the dip – make a well in the mash and then spoon in the muhammara.

This dip keeps well in an airtight container in the refrigerator for around 3–4 days.

LONGEVITY 6 LARDER

MAKES ABOUT 20*

(*depending on size cut)

These crackers are made with a combination of different seeds, providing omega-3 and omega-6 fatty acids, which help keep our blood vessels healthy. Za'atar originates from the Arabic word for 'thyme', one of its main ingredients, often blended with sumac and sesame seeds.

za'atar and sesame seed crackers

- 125g/4½oz sunflower seeds
- 125g/4½oz pumpkin seeds
- 100g/3½oz chia seeds
- 100g/3½oz golden linseeds/flaxseeds
- 25g/1oz sesame seeds
- 2 tsp flaked sea salt
- 4 tsp za'atar
- 240ml/8½fl oz warm water

1. Preheat the oven to 170°C fan/375°F/Gas 5. Line a large baking tray with baking paper.

2. Place all of the ingredients, apart from the za'atar and water, in a large bowl and mix to combine. Scoop out a cupful (about 200g/7oz) and add this to a food processor (or a Nutribullet, if you have one). Blitz to form a powder and then return this to the large bowl. Add the za'atar, stir in the warm water and then set aside for 10 minutes, to thicken slightly.

3. Tip out onto the lined baking tray and, using the back of a spoon, spread out to cover the tray to form a rectangle, about 35 x 30cm/14 x 12in wide and 0.5cm/¼in thick. If it helps, place a sheet of baking paper on top of the mixture and use a rolling pin to roll it out. Either way, before going in the oven, slice how you'd like the crackers to be – rectangles, squares or triangles all work well. Use a pizza cutter if you have one, or a large, sharp knife.

4. Bake for about 35 minutes, rotating the tray halfway through, until crisp and golden.

5. Remove from the oven, then set aside to firm up and cool completely on the baking tray before serving or storing. Serve with the Muhammara (see p.154) or other dips.

COOK'S NOTE

These crackers keep in an airtight container at room temperature for up to a week.

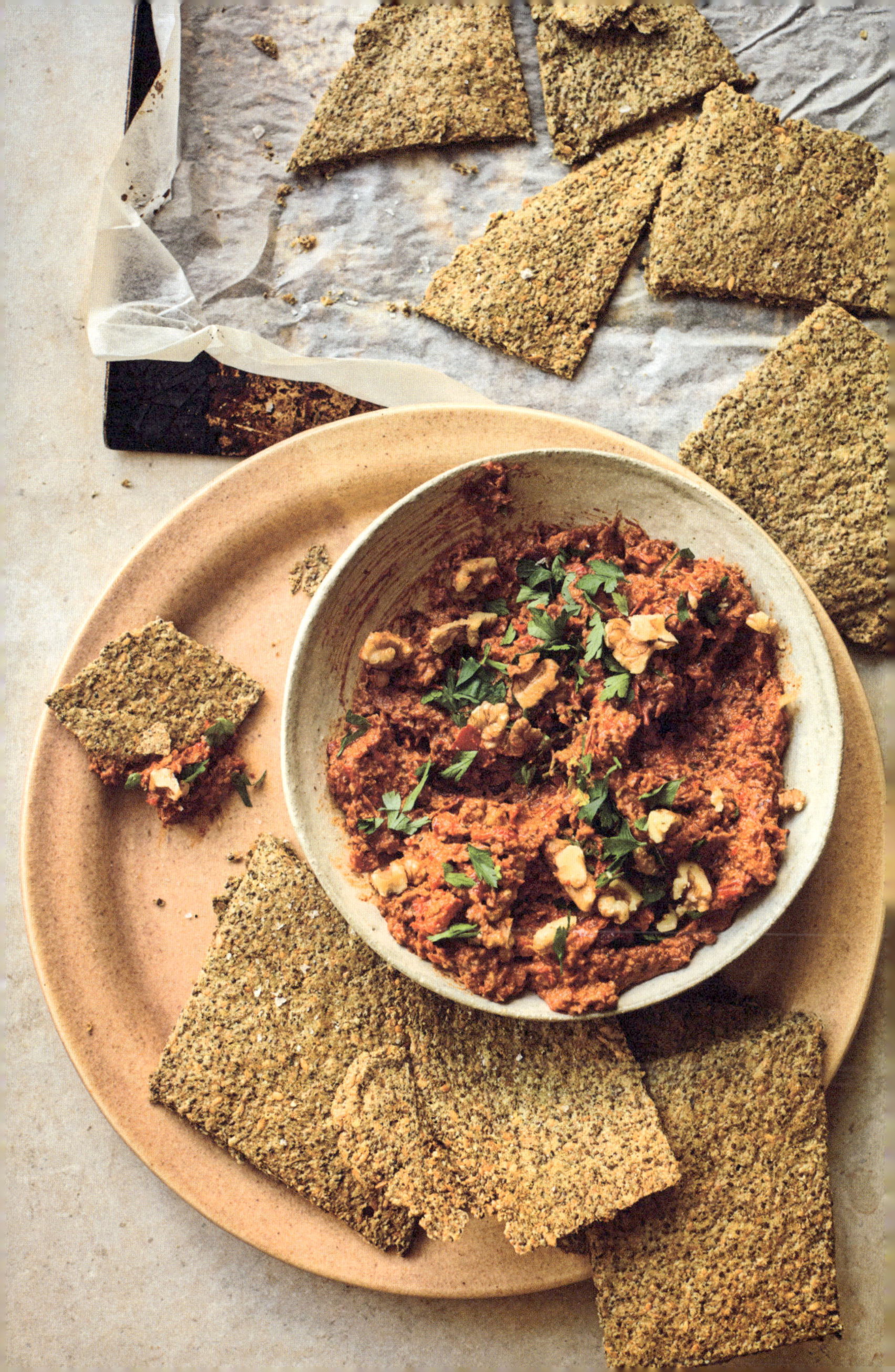

LONGEVITY 15 LARDER

SERVES 4

A super-simple and deliciously nourishing dish – plant-based food at its best, as far as I'm concerned. Opt for skin-roasted peanuts if you can, because a recent clinical trial found that just 25g/1oz a day of skin-roasted peanuts helped preserve telomere length (see pp.19–20), due to the polyphenols, fibre and antioxidants in the skin (which is otherwise stripped away in processing).[114]

tomato, tofu and green bean laksa

- 4 banana shallots, roughly chopped
- 4 garlic cloves, roughly chopped
- 30g/1oz fresh ginger, peeled and roughly chopped
- 2 lemongrass stalks, roughly bruised with a rolling pin, outer leaves discarded, white parts sliced
- 2 tsp ground coriander
- 1 red chilli, deseeded and roughly chopped (optional)
- 2 tbsp sambal oelek
- 1 tbsp maple syrup (or runny honey)
- 20g/¾oz fresh coriander stems, roughly chopped (save the leaves to serve – see below)
- 4 tbsp rapeseed (or other neutral) oil
- 200g/7oz dried flat rice noodles
- 300g/10½oz silken tofu, drained and carefully cut into 2cm/¾in dice
- 1.2 litres/2 pints hot vegetable (or chicken) stock
- 1 tbsp mild curry powder
- 1 x 400ml/14fl oz can coconut milk
- 300g/10½oz cherry tomatoes, halved
- 200g/7oz French beans, trimmed
- Salt

1. Add the first nine ingredients to a blender or Nutribullet, along with 2 tablespoons of the oil and 1 teaspoon of salt. Blitz to form a rough paste.

2. Heat the remaining 2 tablespoons of oil in a large saucepan over a medium-high heat. Add the paste, reduce the heat to medium and cook for 10 minutes, stirring often.

3. Meanwhile, cook the noodles according to the packet instructions, then drain and divide between four bowls. Divide the tofu between the bowls, sitting it on top of the noodles.

4. Add the stock, curry powder and coconut milk to the saucepan and bring to a simmer. Cook for about 10 minutes and then add the tomatoes. Cook for another 5 minutes, then add the French beans and cook for a final 5 minutes.

5. Ladle the laksa into the bowls over the tofu and noodles, then serve with the coriander, mint and peanuts sprinkled on top, along with a lime half on the side of each portion.

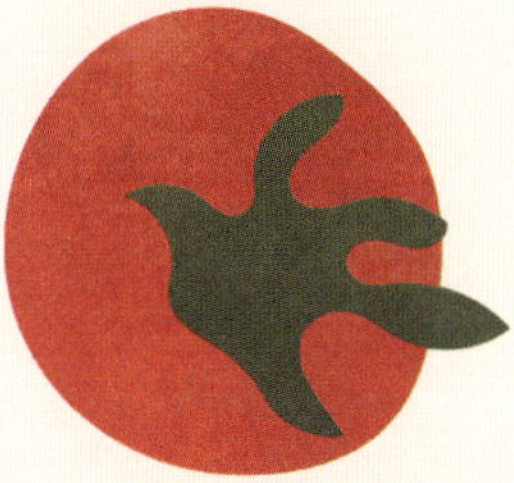

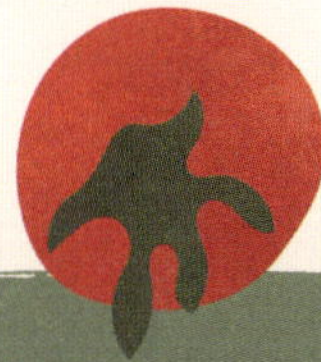

TO SERVE

15g/½oz fresh coriander leaves, chopped
15g/½oz fresh mint leaves, shredded
40g/1½oz peanuts (skin on, if possible) or cashews, lightly toasted (see Cook's Note on p.182) and roughly chopped
2 limes, halved

COOK'S NOTES

Once the laksa base is made, you can mix and match what you want to put into your bowl to serve – everyone can make up their own bowl with all sorts of veg, such as beansprouts and button mushrooms, or another protein source instead of the tofu, suh as cooked prawns or chicken – simply add them in (instead of the French beans) for the final 5 minutes of cooking time. Courgette spaghetti (courgetti) is also an alternative to the noodles.

The laksa base can be made ahead of time (then cook the noodles and assemble the tofu in bowls just before serving). Once made and cooled, it will keep in an airtight container in the refrigerator for up to 3 days, or it can be frozen in portions for up to 2 months, for a ready-made bowl. Reheat gently until piping hot before serving (defrost, if frozen, before reheating).

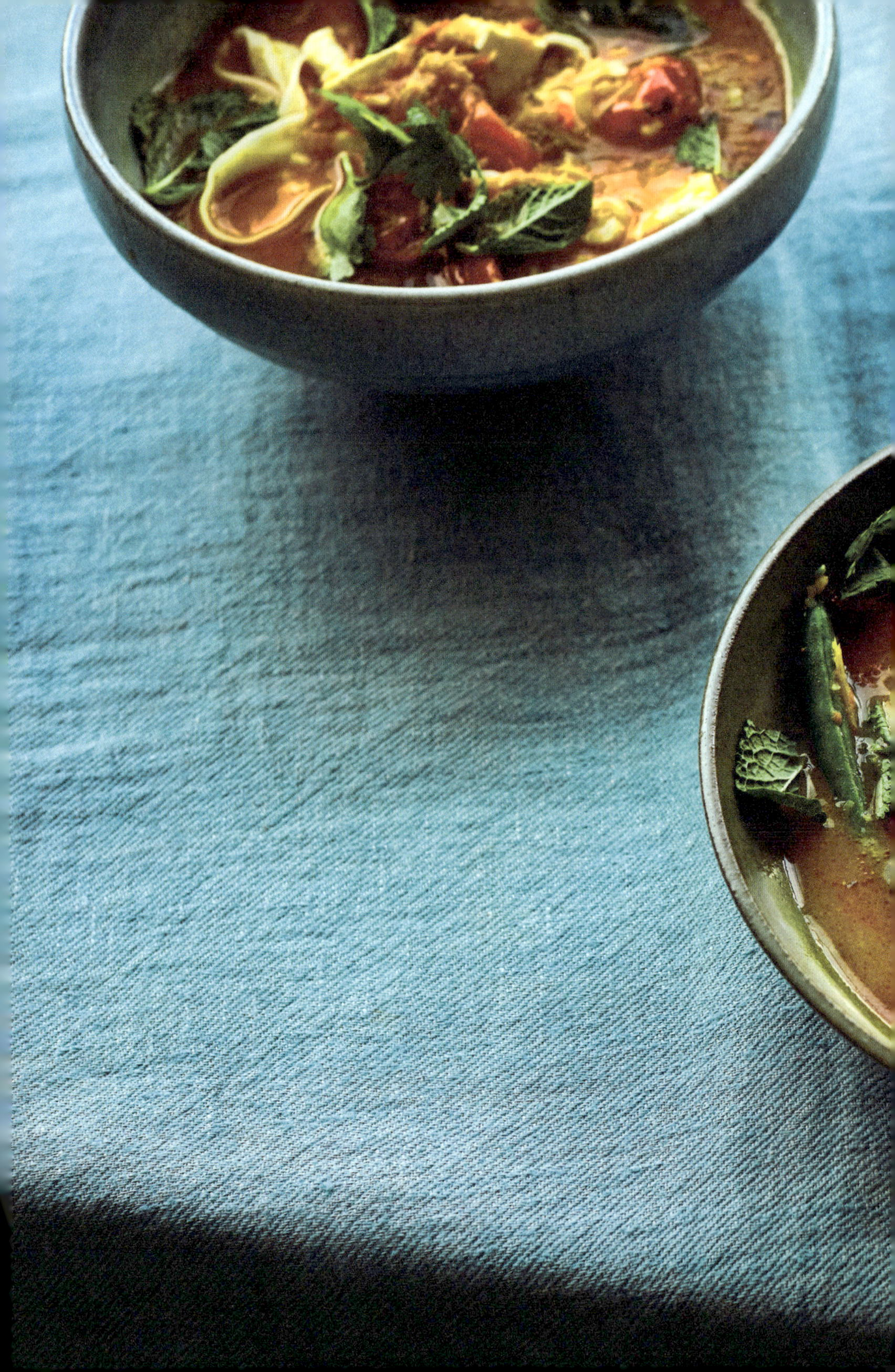

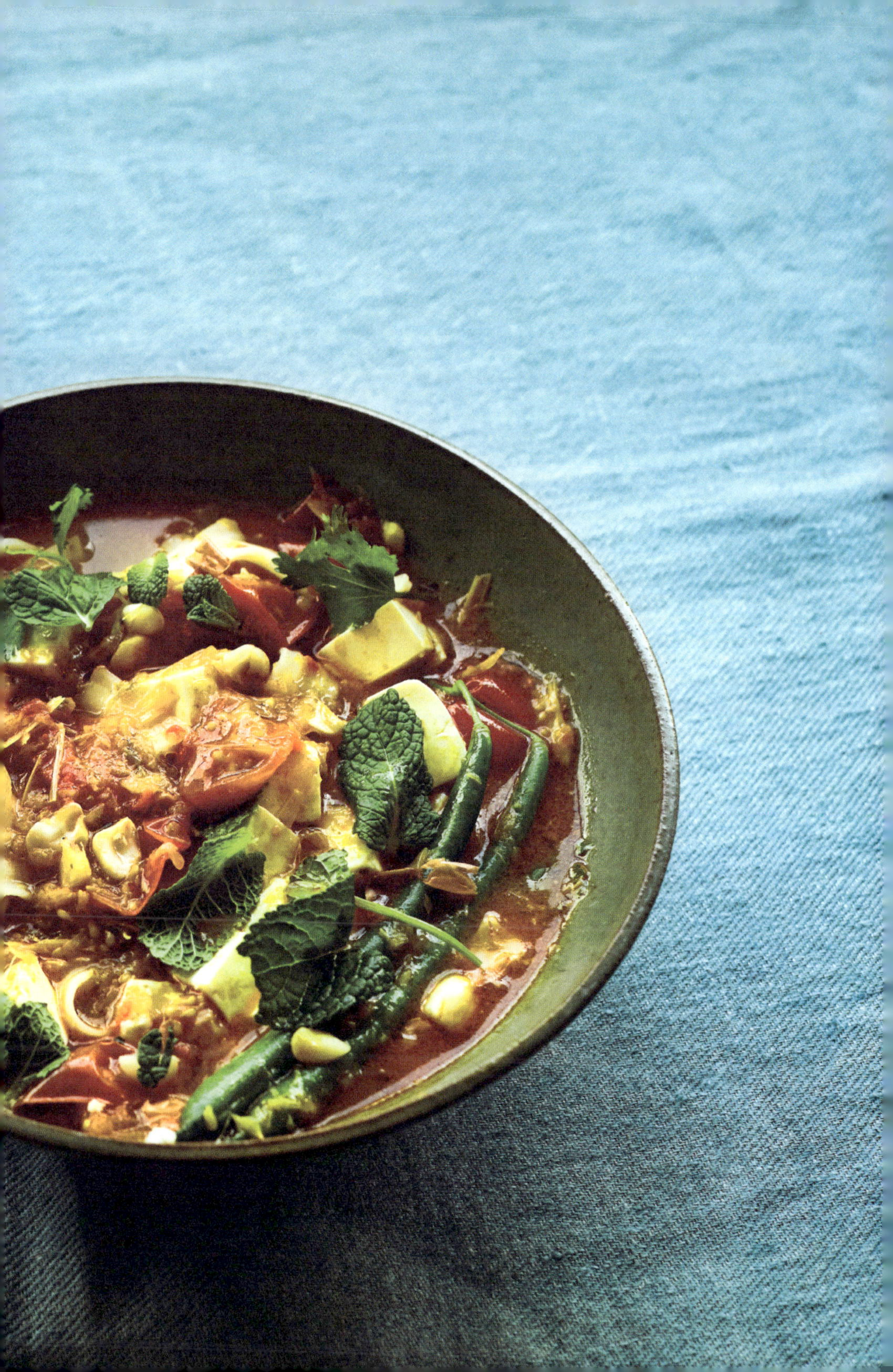

LONGEVITY 13 LARDER

SERVES 4

This rustic Provençal dish takes its name from the Occitan (native to southern France and related to Catalan) *ratatolha*, meaning 'to stir'. It originally included whatever leftover summer vegetables were on offer, often simmered for hours to intensify the flavours. It is a humble dish that is packed full of antioxidants and fibre – here with the bonus addition of some cod and a parsley dressing topper.

oven-baked ratatouille with cod loins and parsley dressing

3 medium-large aubergines, cut into 3–4cm/1¼–1½in dice
3 peppers (a mix of red, yellow and orange looks great), deseeded and cut into 3cm/1¼in dice
2 onions (red or white), cut into 3cm/1¼in chunks
3 courgettes, halved lengthways and cut into 2cm/¾in chunks
2 large garlic cloves, crushed
2 tbsp roughly chopped fresh thyme leaves
2 bay leaves
2 tbsp lemon juice
120ml/4fl oz olive oil
80g/3oz Kalamata olives, pitted and halved
4 skinless cod loins (each about 130–140g/4¾–5oz)
Salt and black pepper

TOMATO SAUCE

1½ tbsp olive oil
2 large garlic cloves, finely sliced
2 x 400g/14oz cans chopped tomatoes
2 sprigs of fresh thyme
1 bay leaf
100ml/3½fl oz water

1. Preheat the oven to 220°C fan/475°F/Gas 9. Line two large baking trays with baking paper.

2. Add the first nine ingredients for the ratatouille to a large mixing bowl, along with a pinch of salt and a good grind of black pepper. Stir well to combine and then spread out on the lined baking trays. Roast for 45 minutes, stirring gently every 15 minutes or so.

3. After 45 minutes, combine all the vegetables onto one tray, reduce the oven temperature to 200°C fan/425°F/Gas 7 and cook for a final 15 minutes. The vegetables should be well cooked and starting to go jammy but not have collapsed altogether. Remove from the oven and set aside.

4. Meanwhile, make the tomato sauce. Add the olive oil to a large sauté pan or casserole pot and place over a medium heat. Add the garlic, cook for just a minute and then add the tomatoes, thyme and bay leaf. Add the water, bring to a simmer and cook for about 30 minutes, covered, stirring a few times, until the sauce has thickened.

PARSLEY DRESSING
30g/1oz fresh parsley leaves, finely chopped
1 garlic clove, crushed
3 tbsp olive oil
1 tbsp lemon juice
Salt and black pepper

5. Lift out and discard the thyme and bay leaf, tip in the roasted vegetables, add the olives and stir gently to combine. Lower in the cod – it wants to be nearly submerged, but not completely – and return the pan to a medium heat. Cover and cook for about 10 minutes (timing will depend on the thickness of the fish), until the fish is just cooked through.

6. Place all of the ingredients for the parsley dressing in the small bowl of a food processor, along with a pinch of salt and a good grind of black pepper. Blitz to combine. Spoon a generous tablespoon of the parsley dressing over each piece of cod and serve straight from the pan.

COOK'S NOTES

Use a mix of veg – whatever you have or what's in season; you'll need about 1.8kg/4lb in total. Cubes of sweet potato, butternut squash or kohlrabi all work well.

This dish can also be a side to roasted chicken, or served on top of cooked brown rice, buckwheat or quinoa. It's also good piled on top of a slice of toasted sourdough (smashed avocado is also lovely on the toast before the ratatouille goes on), or for breakfast with a poached egg on top. It's also delicious served at room temperature!

The parsley dressing is lovely on top, but the dish is also great without it. You can also play around with the herbs – basil or coriander both work well.

Make the full batch of ratatouille, even if you're only feeding one or two, as it keeps (and also freezes) well and leftovers are great to have on hand. It will keep in an airtight container in the refrigerator for up to 3 days, and freezes for up to 2 months. Reheat gently until piping hot before serving (defrost, if frozen, before reheating).

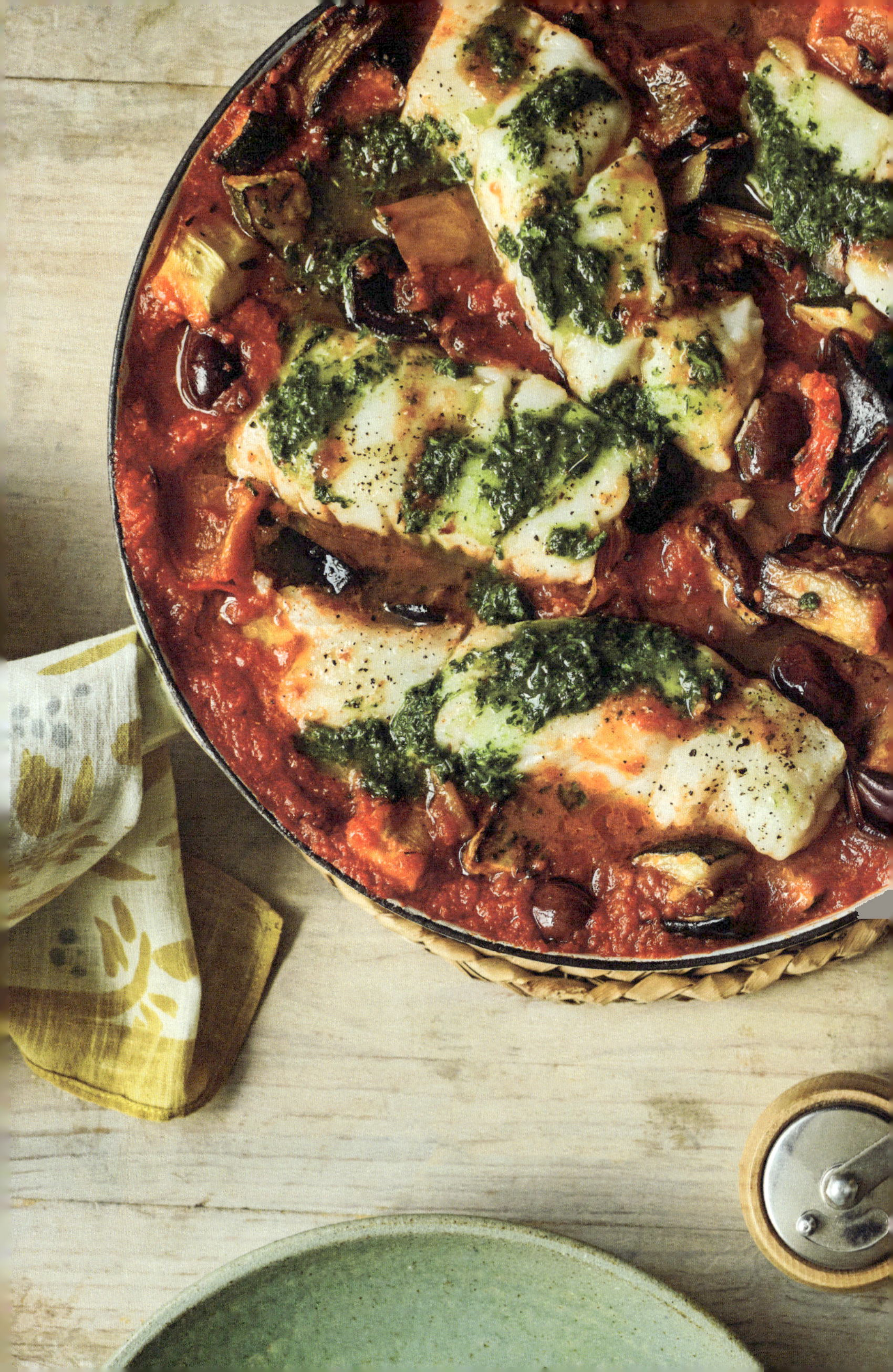

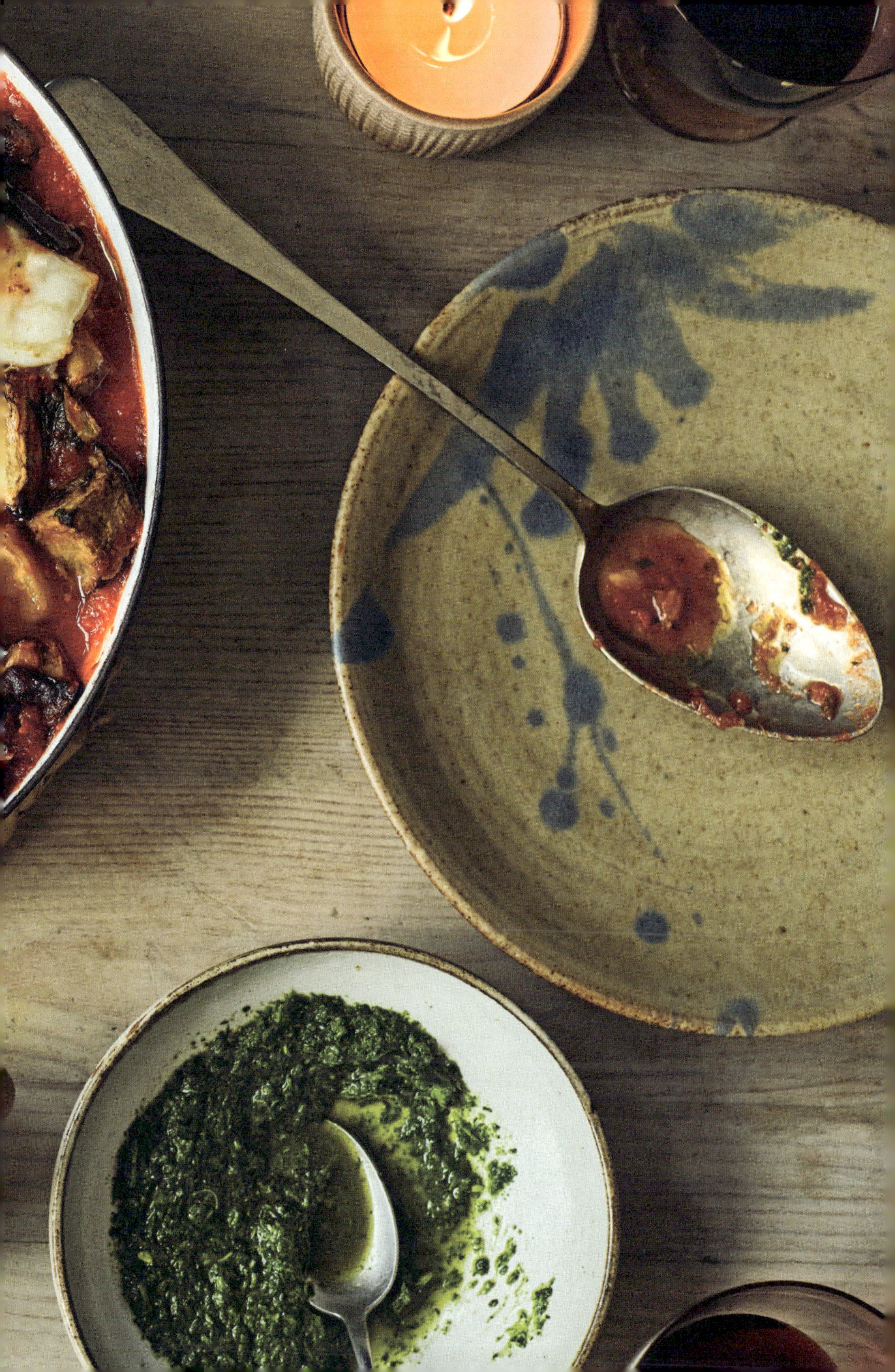

LONGEVITY 14 LARDER

SERVES 4-6

Beany curries like this one give us loads of easy-to-digest protein, plentiful amounts of fibre to help support healthy cholesterol levels, and antioxidants from all the spices and the coriander, which also provides terpinene, quercetin and tocopherol (a form of vitamin E). Butter beans are also a valuable source of iron and folate, as well as potassium, which helps support blood-pressure regulation.

butter bean masala

300g/10½oz large plum or vine tomatoes, quartered lengthways
1 tsp cumin seeds, lightly toasted
5 tbsp olive oil
150g/5½oz cherry tomatoes
4 garlic cloves, roughly chopped
1 tbsp coriander seeds, lightly toasted
25g/1oz fresh ginger, peeled and roughly chopped
30g /1oz fresh coriander, stems roughly chopped (save the leaves – see below)
2 green chillies, roughly chopped (deseeded if preferred)
2 tsp garam masala
1 tsp ground turmeric
1 large onion, thinly sliced
2 x 570g/1lb 4½oz jars butter beans, drained and rinsed
1 x 160ml/5¼fl oz can coconut cream
120g/4¼oz spinach leaves
Salt and black pepper
Fresh coriander leaves (from above), roughly chopped, to garnish

TO SERVE (ANY OR ALL OF THE FOLLOWING)
Natural (or coconut) yogurt
Naan bread or brown rice
Toasted flaked almonds

1. Preheat the oven to 200°C fan/425°F/Gas 7. Line a baking tray with baking paper.

2. In a bowl, mix the large tomatoes with the cumin seeds, 1½ tablespoons of the olive oil, a pinch of salt and a good grind of black pepper. Spread out on the lined baking tray and roast for 10 minutes. Tip in the cherry tomatoes, stir to combine and roast for another 20 minutes, until soft and starting to colour.

3. Meanwhile, add the garlic, coriander seeds, ginger, coriander stems, chillies, garam masala and turmeric to the small bowl of a food processor (or blender), along with 2 tablespoons of the olive oil and 2 teaspoons of salt. Blitz to form a rough paste.

4. Add the remaining 1½ tablespoons of olive oil to a large sauté pan or saucepan and place over a medium-high heat. Add the onion and cook for about 6 minutes, stirring from time to time, until soft and starting to caramelize. Add the spice paste and continue to cook for another 6 minutes, stirring and adding a good splash of water if needed.

5. Tip in the roasted tomatoes and cook for 3–4 minutes, stirring to combine and mashing up some of the tomatoes. Add the butter beans, coconut cream and spinach. Cook for another couple of minutes, enough for the spinach to wilt.

6. Serve the butter bean masala with the coriander leaves sprinkled on top to garnish. Add a spoonful of yogurt alongside and any of the other extras – the naan or rice and/or the flaked almonds – as desired.

COOK'S NOTES

If there are any leftovers, cool, then store them in an airtight container in the refrigerator for up to 3 days. Reheat gently in a pan until piping hot before serving.

For serving, the Coriander–Walnut Pesto for the Red Lentil and Harissa Soup (see p.172) also works well here, as does the Kale and Almond Pesto in the Pearl Barley and Brothy Bean Soup (see p.134), but just the coriander leaves as they are, are also enough.

clarity tonic

nutty blueberry porridge

red lentil and harissa soup with coriander–walnut pesto

pan-fried salmon with white beans, charred tomatoes and salsa verde

yellow thai curry

tash's thai salad

berry crumble with roasted plum yogurt

brain food

LONGEVITY 6 LARDER

SERVES 2

This brain-supporting tonic includes beetroot for nitric oxide, to help get oxygen to the brain, alongside blueberries and acai for their anthocyanins, beta carotene-rich carrots and vitamin C from the lemon. Celery is from the family of 'nervines', which have been used in herbal medicine to help calm the nervous system.

clarity tonic

2 fresh beetroots (no need to peel)
80g/3oz fresh blueberries
3 carrots (no need to peel)
3 celery sticks
1 lemon, peeled and roughly chopped
1 tsp acai powder (optional)

1. Wash the first four ingredients, then chop them to fit into your juicer. Add the lemon, and juice.

2. Stir the acai powder (if using) into your finished juice, then pour into glasses and enjoy.

LONGEVITY 9 LARDER

SERVES 1

Time to add more brain-loving ingredients to the humble porridge, and more protein sources to help sustain a drip feed of energy across your morning to boost your mood. This is a great way to get your nut intake in at breakfast, as well as supporting your second brain, the gut, with the beta glucan-rich oats and ground linseed/flaxseed.

nutty blueberry porridge

- 40g/1½oz rolled oats or jumbo oats
- 1 tbsp ground linseed/flaxseed
- 1 tbsp pumpkin seeds
- 1 tbsp hemp seeds
- 1 tbsp chia seeds
- 1 tbsp chopped walnuts
- ½ tsp ground cinnamon or ground cardamom (or both!)
- 80g/3oz frozen blueberries (frozen cherries also work well)
- 200ml/7fl oz milk of your choice

TOPPINGS (ONE OR BOTH OF THE FOLLOWING)

- 1 tbsp almond butter
- 2 tbsp Greek-style, soy or coconut yogurt

1. Pop all the porridge ingredients in a small saucepan and slowly bring to a simmer. Gently simmer for around 3–4 minutes, stirring occasionally, until the blueberries become squishy.

2. Serve in a bowl with the nut butter on top and/or the yogurt.

LONGEVITY 12 LARDER

SERVES 4*

(*with leftover pesto)

A most delicious plant-based soup, with lentils as a great source of plant-based iron (to help get more oxygen to the brain in order to reduce brain fatigue), folate to support neurotransmitter production, and a whole host of spices for their antioxidants. Tomatoes also provide antioxidant lycopene, and there's limonene in the lemon zest (do make sure you buy unwaxed lemons).

red lentil and harissa soup with coriander–walnut pesto

- 2 tbsp olive oil, plus extra for drizzling to serve
- 2 onions, finely chopped
- 2 large garlic cloves, crushed
- 1 large carrot, peeled and cut into 1cm/½in dice
- 20g/¾oz fresh coriander stems, finely chopped
- 2 tsp ground cumin
- 2 tsp ground coriander
- 2 tbsp rose harissa
- 2 tbsp tomato purée
- 250g/9oz dried whole red lentils, rinsed and drained
- 1 x 400g/14oz can chopped tomatoes
- About 1 litre/1¾ pints vegetable stock
- 1 lemon, quartered, to serve (zest it for the pesto before slicing)

1. Place all the ingredients for the pesto (see overleaf) in a food processor along with 1 teaspoon of salt and a good grind of black pepper. Blitz to form a coarse paste and set aside.

2. Make the soup. Add the olive oil to a medium saucepan and place over a medium heat. Add the onions and cook for about 8 minutes, stirring from time to time, until softened and taking on some colour.

3. Add the garlic, carrot and coriander stems and cook for another 5 minutes, before adding the ground spices, harissa and tomato purée. Cook for another minute or two, stirring, before adding the lentils, tomatoes and stock. Give everything a good stir, then bring to a simmer and cook, partially covered, for about 20 minutes, stirring a few times.

recipe continues overleaf

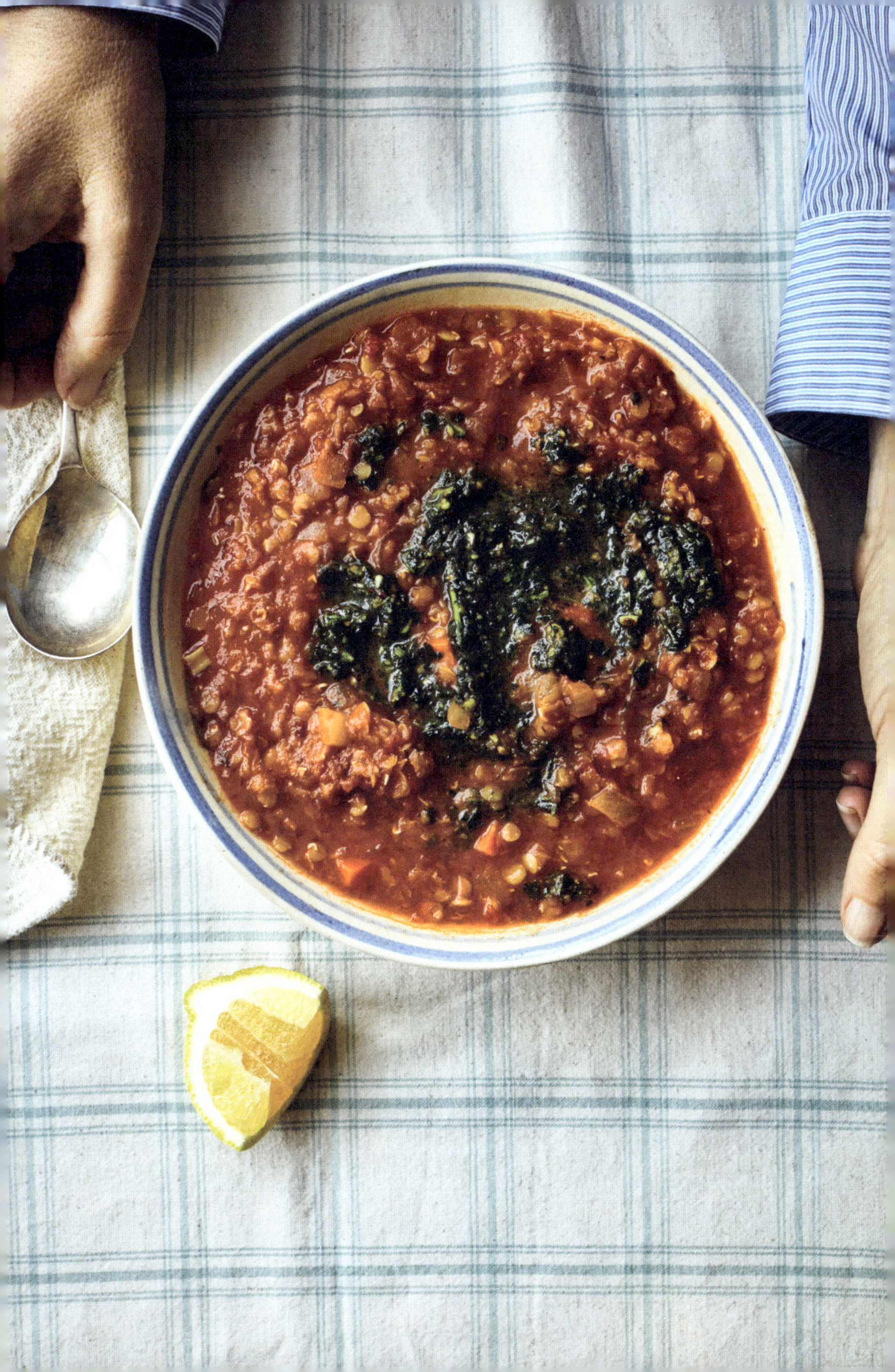

CORIANDER–WALNUT PESTO

80g/3oz fresh coriander, roughly chopped
60g/2¼oz walnuts, lightly toasted (see Cook's Note on p.182) and roughly chopped
1½ tsp coriander seeds, lightly toasted and roughly crushed
Finely grated zest of 1 lemon (use lemon from above)
1 garlic clove, crushed
100ml/3½fl oz olive oil
Salt and black pepper

4. You now have the option either to blitz the soup until smooth or leave it as it is and serve (I prefer to leave it as it is as I like a chunkier soup). Either way, ladle it into bowls, swirl a spoonful of the pesto through each portion (you won't need all the pesto – see Cook's Notes below) and serve with a final drizzle of olive oil on top and a wedge of lemon alongside.

COOK'S NOTES

Store leftover pesto in an airtight container/jar in the refrigerator for up to 4 days, or freeze for up to 2 months (defrost before use).

The Coriander–Walnut Pesto also works well with the Roasted Ginger and Coconut Tomatoes with White Beans and Sea Bass on p.138.

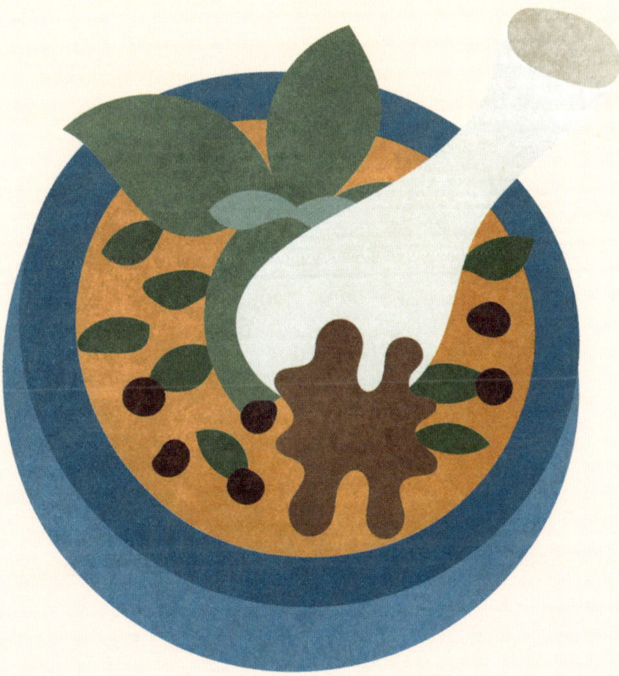

LONGEVITY 13 LARDER

SERVES 2*

(*with leftover salsa verde)

An incredibly simple dish with a very Mediterranean feel. It provides nervous-system support from the omega-3s in the salmon, as well as all the essential amino acids. The olive oil in the salsa verde helps the absorption of the beta carotene coming from the herbs, as this antioxidant needs fat to be digested. Alongside all of this are cannellini beans, to help feed the microbiome – our second brain.

pan-fried salmon with white beans, charred tomatoes and salsa verde

3 tbsp olive oil
200g/7oz cherry tomatoes
2 salmon fillets, skin on (each about 170g/6oz)
2 large banana shallots, finely chopped
1 x 400g/14oz can cannellini beans, drained (but keep hold of the liquid) and rinsed
50g/1¾oz crème fraîche (optional)
Salt and black pepper

SALSA VERDE
10g/¼oz fresh mint leaves
10g/¼oz fresh basil leaves
10g/¼oz fresh parsley leaves
10g/¼oz fresh tarragon leaves
40g/1½oz capers, drained
2 tsp Dijon mustard
2 garlic cloves, roughly chopped
15g/½oz canned anchovy fillets in oil (5–7 fillets, depending on size), drained
2 tbsp sherry or red wine vinegar
4 tbsp olive oil

1. Place all of the ingredients for the salsa verde in a food processor and pulse a few times, to form a coarse paste. Transfer to a clean sealed jar and keep in the refrigerator until ready to use.

2. Add 1 teaspoon of the olive oil to a large frying pan and place over a high heat. Once hot, add the tomatoes, along with a pinch of salt. Cook for about 5 minutes, shaking the pan a few times, until charred and just beginning to collapse. Remove from the pan to a plate and set aside.

3. Return the pan to a medium-high heat and add 2 more teaspoons of the olive oil. Once hot, add the salmon, skin-side down, and pan-fry for about 7 minutes (timing will depend on the thickness of the fillets), turning so that all sides take on some colour and the fish is cooked through. Transfer to a plate and set aside at room temperature (or keep warm, if preferred) until serving.

4. Wipe the pan clean, then add the remaining 2 tablespoons of olive oil and place over a medium heat. Add the shallots and a pinch of salt, then cook for about 8 minutes, stirring often and adding a splash of liquid from the beans (or water or white wine, if handy), until soft. Add the beans, along with another splash of their liquid and a good grind of black pepper and stir through for 2–3 minutes. Add the crème fraîche (if using) and stir to combine.

5. Divide the bean mixture between two plates. Swirl a generous portion of the salsa verde through each portion of beans (there will be leftover salsa verde – see Cook's Notes below), top with the salmon and charred tomatoes and serve.

COOK'S NOTES

The salsa verde will make twice as much as you need, but it keeps well in the refrigerator for up to 4 days or so and is great with all sorts of things: any cooked fish or chicken, in a sandwich or wrap, or drizzled over fried or poached eggs. It's a great way of using up herbs, too!

You can make this vegetarian by removing the anchovies from the salsa verde (just up the capers), and instead of the fish, serving the creamy beans, charred tomatoes and salsa verde with some pan-fried halloumi or cubes of fresh feta cheese. Serve with a rocket or other green salad.

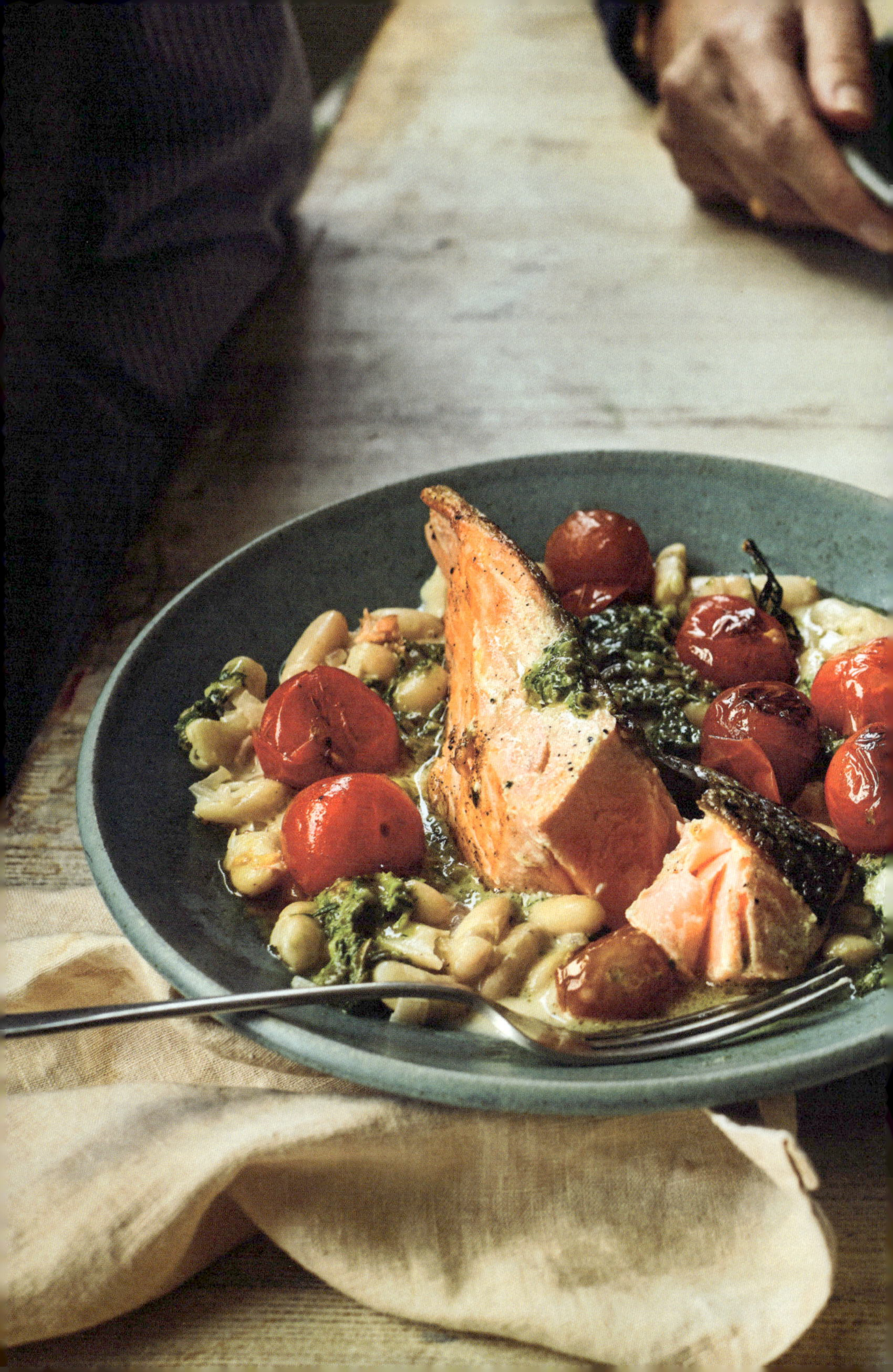

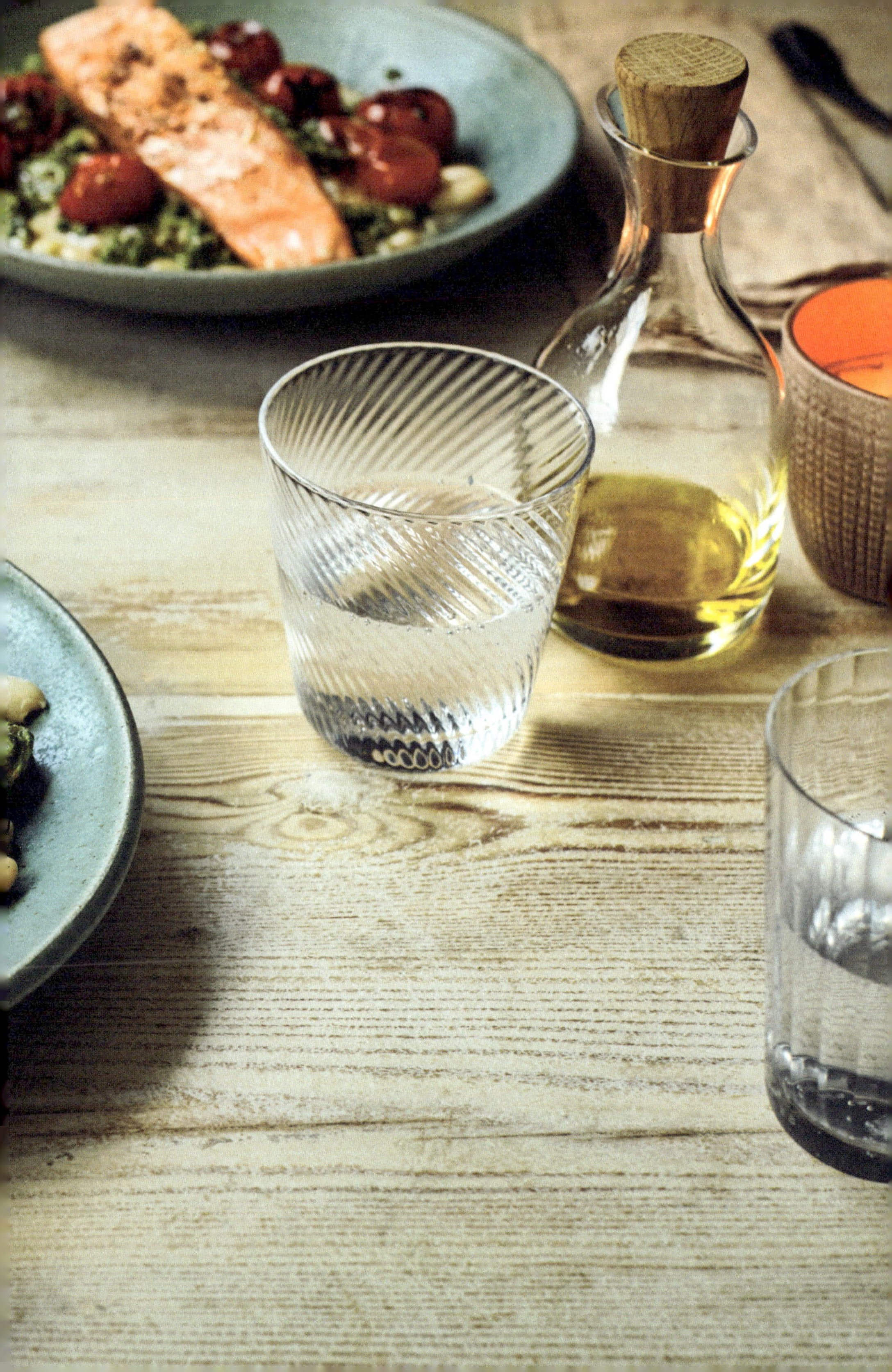

LONGEVITY 16 LARDER

SERVES 4

Peppers are a brilliant source of vitamin C, shallots are a great source of nature's antihistamine and antioxidant quercetin, and turmeric and ginger both provide potent anti-inflammatory qualities. Packed full of antioxidant-rich herbs and spices, too, like a lot of Thai food, which is why I love it so much! You can use no-fish 'fish' sauce to make this vegan, if preferred.

yellow thai curry

CURRY BASE

2 peppers (yellow or red or a mixture), deseeded and cut into 3cm/1¼in chunks
1 large yellow or green courgette, sliced lengthways and then into half-moons, 1.5cm/⅝in-thick
120g/4¼oz button or chestnut mushrooms, halved or quartered
100g/3½oz baby corn, sliced in half lengthways
1 tsp ground turmeric
3 tbsp olive oil
1 x 400ml/14fl oz can coconut milk
1 x 160ml/5¼fl oz can coconut cream
1 tbsp Thai fish sauce
1 tbsp maple syrup (or soft light brown sugar)
Salt and black pepper

1. Preheat the oven to 220°C fan/475°F/Gas 9. Line a baking tray with baking paper.

2. In a large bowl, mix together the peppers, courgette, mushrooms, baby corn, turmeric and olive oil, along with ½ teaspoon of salt and a good grind of black pepper. Spread out on the lined baking tray and roast for about 20 minutes, stirring halfway through, for everything to soften and take on some colour. Remove from the oven and set aside.

3. Place all the ingredients for the spice paste (see overleaf) in a blender, along with 4 tablespoons of the coconut milk and 1 tablespoon of the coconut cream from the curry base ingredients list (left). Blitz to make a paste.

4. Add the remaining coconut cream to a large saucepan or sauté pan and place over a medium heat. Bring to a simmer and then add the spice paste. Cook for about 10 minutes, stirring frequently; it will start to look oily and begin to separate but this is how it should be.

recipe continues overleaf

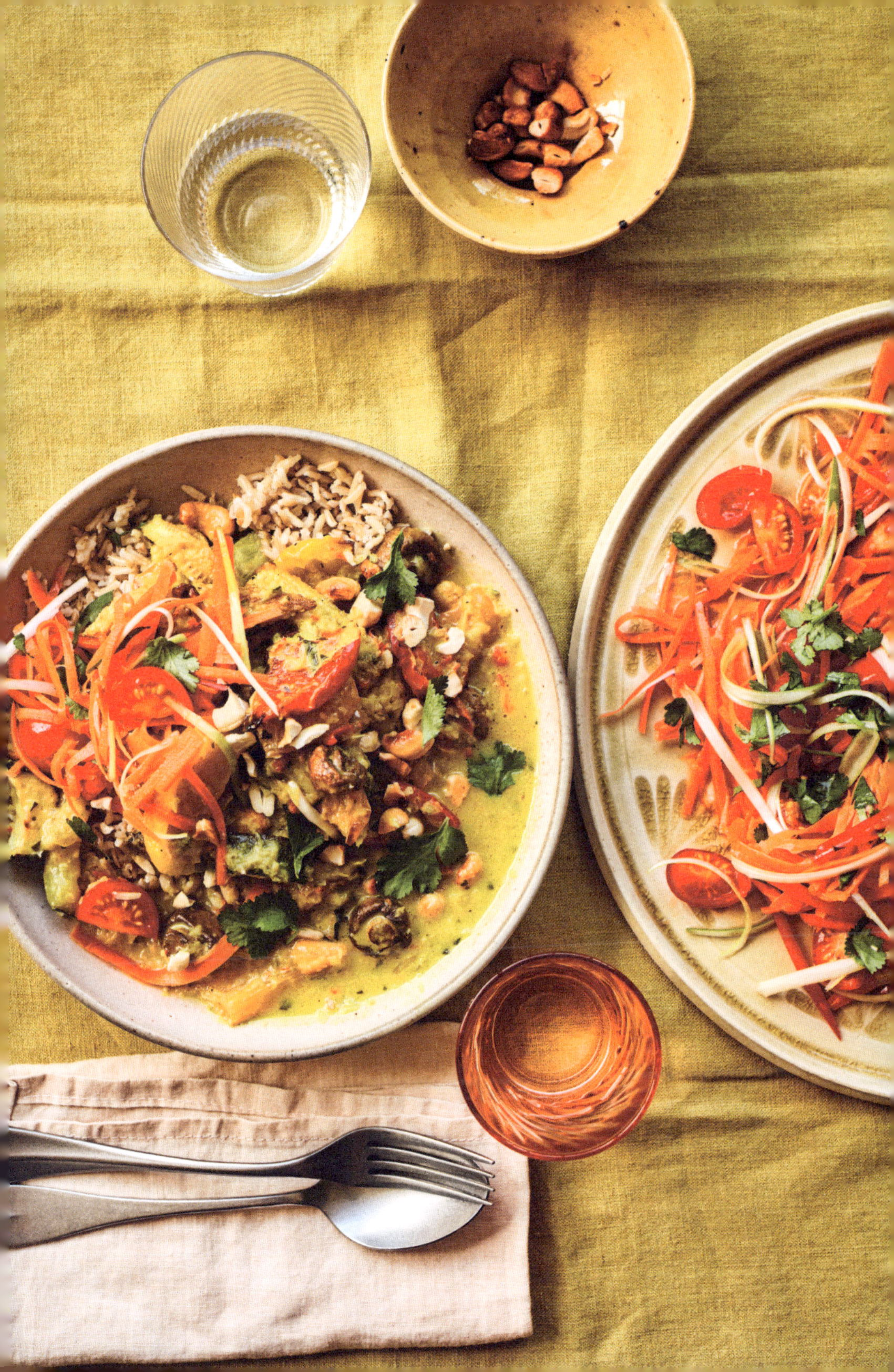

SPICE PASTE

2–3 banana shallots, roughly chopped
2 garlic cloves, roughly chopped
10g/¼oz fresh ginger, peeled and roughly chopped
1 red chilli, deseeded and roughly chopped
4 makrut lime leaves (ideally fresh, but dried are fine too)
½ tsp ground turmeric
1 tsp ground coriander
½ tsp salt
20g/¾oz fresh coriander, stems only (keep the leaves to serve – see below)

TO SERVE

Plain white jasmine or brown rice are both great (or sticky rice and prawn crackers, if you prefer)
40g/1½oz cashew nuts, toasted (see Cook's Notes) and roughly chopped
Fresh coriander leaves (from above)

5. Add the remaining coconut milk, the fish sauce and maple syrup and bring to a simmer. Cook for about 5 minutes, then add the roasted vegetables and warm through for a minute or two.

6. Serve the curry on top of rice, with the toasted cashews and the coriander leaves sprinkled on top.

COOK'S NOTES

To toast nuts, preheat the oven to 160°C fan/350°F/Gas 4. Spread out the nuts on a baking tray and toast in the oven for 8–12 minutes, shaking the tray a couple of times. Cool completely before use. Toasting nuts in the oven like this (rather than in a dry frying pan on the hob) will give you a far more even toast.

Once you have the curry base, you can do what you want in terms of what goes in: cooked prawns and some green beans are great, mangetout or asparagus when in season, cooked chicken thighs (or leftover roast chicken). Also, play around with veggies you have – see it as a bit of a refrigerator raid – you'll need about 700g/1lb 9oz in total. Bear in mind that some veggies – root veggies and things like aubergine – will need longer in the oven at the outset to soften (35–40 minutes), compared to the peppers and courgette.

LONGEVITY
7
LARDER

SERVES
4*
(*as a side)

I love Thai salads because they are so fresh and vibrant, unlike the limp salads I grew up with in the 1980s. I have always loved my friend Tash's creation – Tash is one of my circle of rustle-up friends, who can seamlessly host a whole kitchen full of us without breaking much of a sweat. She was born in Thailand and grew up in Hong Kong, and she always serves this as part of a delicious spread of dishes, often alongside a Thai curry or a lovely barbecued lamb.

tash's thai salad

SALAD
400g/14oz carrots, peeled and julienned
150g/5½oz cherry tomatoes, quartered
3 spring onions, halved and thinly sliced lengthways
25g/1oz fresh coriander leaves, roughly chopped
1 red chilli, deseeded and sliced lengthways

DRESSING
2 tbsp Thai fish sauce
2 tbsp lime juice
2 tsp soft light brown sugar (or 1½ tsp maple syrup)
1 garlic clove, crushed

1. Mix all the salad ingredients together in a salad bowl.
2. Mix all the dressing ingredients together in a small bowl. Pour it over the salad ingredients, toss gently to mix and then leave for an hour or so to marinate in the refrigerator.
3. Serve with the Yellow Thai Curry (see p.180), or try serving it as Tash does, with barbecued lamb.

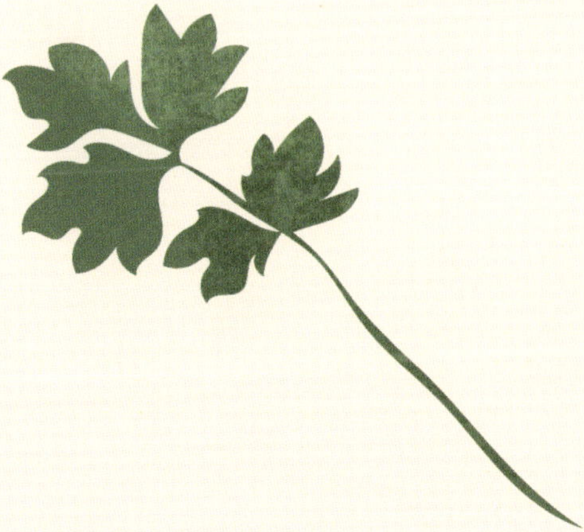

LONGEVITY 15 LARDER

SERVES 4–6

Pudding and breakfast in one! This is delicious warm for pudding, but also good straight from the refrigerator for the next couple of days for breakfast. Strawberries have been shown to modestly improve cognition in older adults,[115] and a greater cumulative total fruit intake (including plums and blueberries) in midlife and later life was significantly associated with a 44 per cent decreased risk of all-cause dementia.[116]

berry crumble with roasted plum yogurt

ROASTED PLUM YOGURT

300g/10½oz plums (ideally purple as they contain more antioxidants), quartered and stoned
2 tbsp maple syrup
10g/¼oz fresh ginger, peeled and grated
½ tsp ground cinnamon
1 tbsp lemon juice
300g/10½oz Greek-style yogurt

FRUIT

400g/14oz frozen berries (I used 200g/7oz blueberries and 200g/7oz strawberries)
100g/3½oz plums (ideally purple – see above), quartered and stoned
½ tsp finely grated orange zest
½ tsp ground cinnamon
¼ tsp ground ginger
1 tbsp cornflour
1 tsp maple syrup
1 tsp acai powder
1 tbsp chia seeds

1. Preheat the oven to 240°C fan/500°F/Gas high (or as close to this as your oven will go). Line a baking tray with baking paper.

2. For the roasted plum yogurt, spread the plums out on the lined baking tray, cut-side up. Roast for 15 minutes, until soft and jammy.

3. Transfer the roasted plums to a food processor, along with the maple syrup, ginger, cinnamon and lemon juice. Blitz well until smooth, then set aside to cool. Once cool, mix with the yogurt in a bowl until combined, then refrigerate until ready to use.

4. Reduce the oven temperature to 170°C fan/375°F/Gas 5.

5. Mix together all the ingredients for the fruit in a 22cm/8½in round (or similar) baking dish and set aside.

recipe continues overleaf

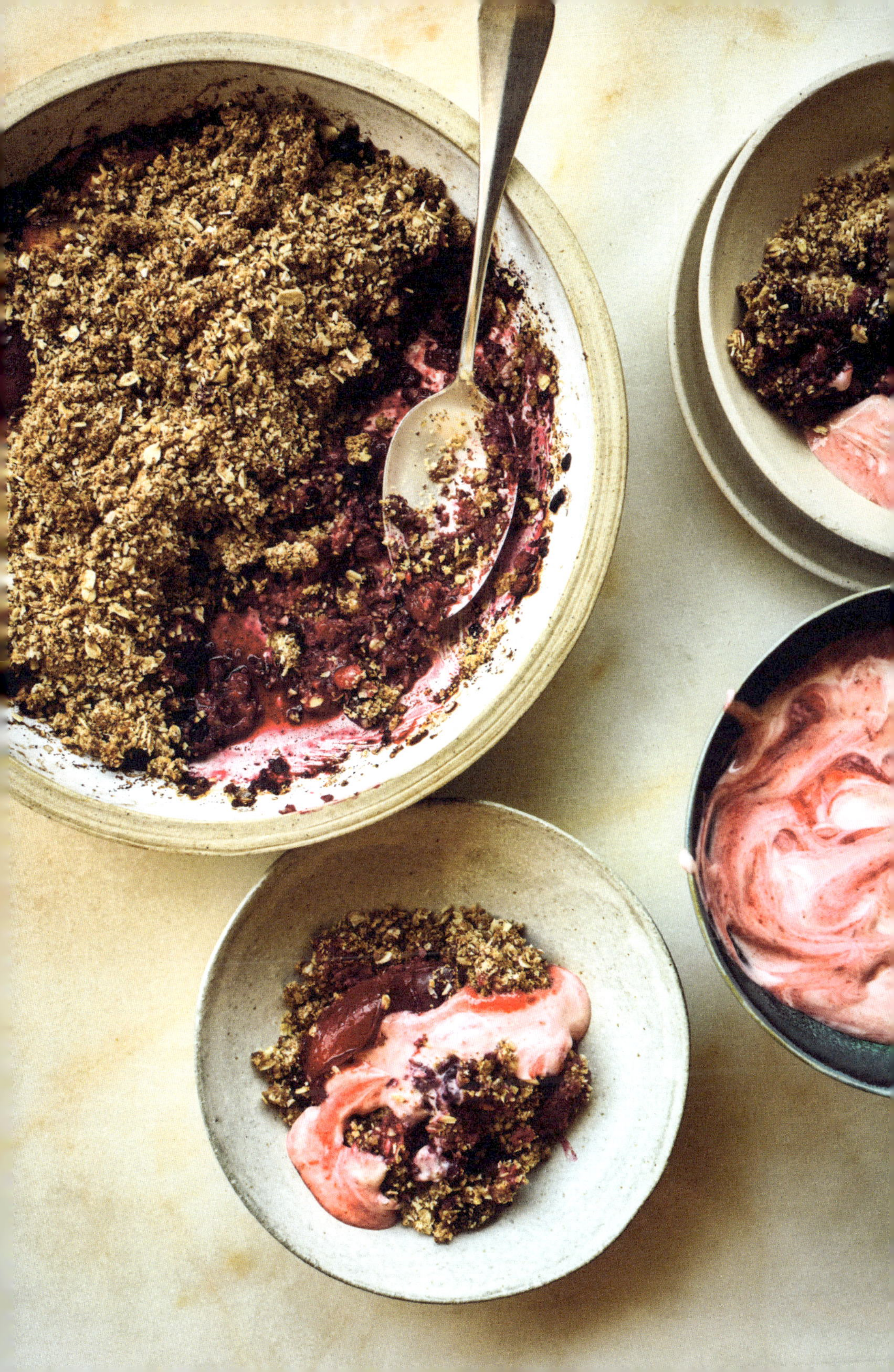

CRUMBLE
120g/4¼oz jumbo oats
4 tbsp almond (or other nut) butter
1 tbsp maple syrup
50g/1¾oz walnuts or pecans
1 tbsp ground linseed/flaxseed
¼ tsp ground cinnamon
Good pinch of ground ginger
2 tsp black (or white) sesame seeds
½ tsp salt

6. Add all the ingredients for the crumble to a food processor and pulse just a few times: you just want to break everything up and combine, rather than be ground too fine. Spread the crumble out on top of the fruit, then bake for 30 minutes, until the top is crisp and golden.

7. Serve the crumble warm with the roasted plum yogurt spooned on top or alongside.

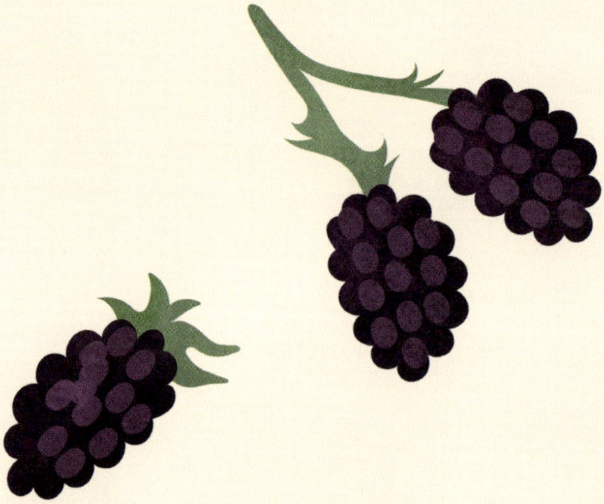

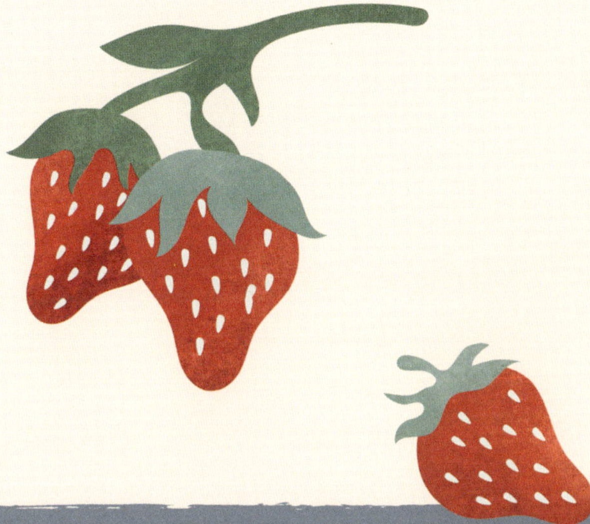

COOK'S NOTES

Roasting the fruit is a great way of ramping up the depth of flavour, making it into a rich compote that can then be stirred through natural yogurt. If you don't want to make the plum yogurt, the crumble is still great with just a spoonful of crème fraîche or thick natural yogurt.

The berries don't need to be frozen but it's a much more economical way of making the crumble. Other fruit options include cooking apple or pear slices, or frozen raspberries, mixed berries or cherries – just keep the net weight (500g/1lb 2oz) about the same.

If there are any leftovers, cool, then store them in an airtight container in the refrigerator for up to 3 days. Warm them through before serving, or eat as is for breakfast!

the unbreakable juice

rose chocolate pots

chipotle chicken traybake with coconut black beans, sweet potato and lime

cauliflower biryani

posh baked beans with feta and kale and almond pesto

hoi an-style chicken and carrot rice

sesame-crusted tofu and herb-packed greens

unbreakable

LONGEVITY 7 LARDER

SERVES 1

This juice is designed to flood your bones with calcium-rich spinach and parsley, alongside magnesium, too. Ginger is there to reduce inflammation, which can affect our bone health, and the lime provides vitamin C for additional antioxidants.

the unbreakable juice

½ cucumber
100g/3½oz spinach leaves
2 large celery sticks
30g/1oz fresh parsley
30g/1oz fresh ginger (no need to peel)
1 eating apple
1 lime, peeled and roughly chopped

1. Wash the everything except the lime, then chop them to fit into your juicer. Add the lime flesh, and juice.

2. Pour into a glass and enjoy.

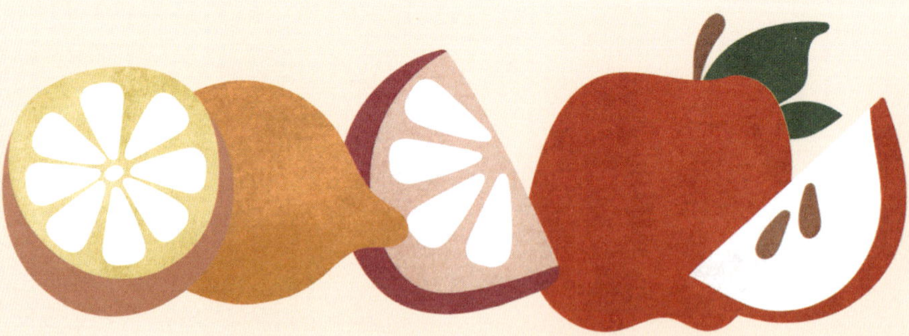

LONGEVITY 6 LARDER

SERVES 4

I love dark chocolate, and it's a bonus that it provides the antioxidant cacao, which is also rich in calcium. This is blended with tofu, which is another great source of calcium, while also providing protein for our bones and isoflavones, which are antioxidants and phytoestrogens.

rose chocolate pots

150g/5½oz dark chocolate (at least 70 per cent cocoa solids), roughly chopped
300g/10½oz silken tofu, drained
1 tbsp rosewater (orange blossom water also works well)
1 tbsp tahini
1 tbsp cacao powder
¼ tsp ground nutmeg
Pinch of salt
Sprinkling of crushed pistachios, to finish

1. Melt the chocolate in a heatproof bowl set over a pan of gently simmering water (be careful not to let the base of the bowl touch the water).

2. Pour the melted chocolate into a food processor and add the silken tofu, rosewater, tahini, cacao powder, nutmeg and the pinch of salt. Blend until smooth.

3. Divide the mixture between four espresso cups, sprinkle on the crushed pistachios (see also Cook's Note) to finish and serve at room temperature – these are best served freshly made.

COOK'S NOTE
Crushed almonds or sesame seeds also work well as a sprinkle to finish.

LONGEVITY LARDER 17

SERVES 4–6

In this traybake, collagen-rich chicken also provides an abundance of minerals, including zinc, selenium, iron (especially the darker cuts), phosphorus and potassium, which are all needed for bone structure and repair. Black beans are also high in minerals such as iron, phosphorus, calcium, magnesium, manganese, copper and zinc. The sweet potato provides the antioxidant beta carotene, and there is plenty of onion here for nature's antihistamine quercetin.

chipotle chicken traybake with coconut black beans, sweet potato and lime

8 chicken thighs, bone in and skin on (about 1kg/2lb 4oz total)
1 tbsp olive oil
½ red onion, roughly chopped
2 large garlic cloves, roughly chopped
2 tsp ground cumin
2 tsp smoked paprika
2 tbsp chipotle chilli paste (Gran Luchito, if possible)
1 tbsp tomato purée
1 x 400ml/14fl oz can coconut milk
1½ tbsp lime juice
100g/3½oz fresh coriander, stems roughly chopped (save the leaves – see below)
2 x 400g/14oz cans black beans, drained and rinsed
1 sweet potato, peeled and cut into 2.5cm/1in chunks
1 red pepper, deseeded and cut into 2.5cm/1in cubes
Salt and black pepper

1. Preheat the oven to 200°C fan/425°F/Gas 7.

2. Place the chicken and olive oil in a bowl with 1 teaspoon of salt and a good grind of black pepper. Mix well to combine and set aside until needed.

3. Place the next nine ingredients in a food processor, along with 1 teaspoon of salt and a good grind of black pepper. Blitz well to combine and then tip into a large baking dish or roasting tray, about 30 x 20cm/12 x 8in. Add the beans, sweet potato, red pepper and the seasoned chicken and mix well, then arrange so that the chicken thighs are skin-side up and poking out slightly. Cover the dish or tray tightly with foil.

4. Bake for 35 minutes and then remove the foil. Bake for another 35 minutes, until everything is well cooked and starting to colour.

5. Meanwhile, make your pickled onion and the sweetcorn salsa, and prepare any extras.

PICKLED ONION
½ red onion, halved and thinly sliced
1 tbsp lime juice
Salt

SWEETCORN SALSA
2 tsp olive oil
2 corn cobs, kernels shaved off, or 200g/7oz frozen corn kernels, defrosted
25g/1oz fresh coriander leaves (from above), roughly chopped
¼ red onion, finely chopped
1½ tbsp lime juice
1 tbsp olive oil
1 red chilli, deseeded and finely chopped (optional)

EXTRAS (ANY OR ALL OF THE FOLLOWING)
Fresh coriander leaves (from above)
Cooked brown rice
Sour cream
Diced avocado
Lime wedges

6. For the pickled onion, add the onion and lime juice to a small bowl with a pinch of salt. Mix well to combine and then set aside to pickle until needed.

7. For the sweetcorn salsa, add the olive oil to a large frying pan and place over a high heat. Once hot, add the corn kernels and fry for 5–6 minutes, stirring regularly, until well charred. Remove from the heat and set aside to cool before mixing through all the remaining salsa ingredients. Keep in a bowl until ready to serve.

8. Remove the chicken traybake from the oven and set aside to rest for 5 minutes. Spoon the pickled onion over the chicken and serve straight from the dish/tray, along with the sweetcorn salsa and any extras that you've prepared.

COOK'S NOTES

You can use chicken legs instead of thighs, if preferred. If you are wanting to use chicken breasts, just make sure they are the chicken supreme cut (i.e. with the little bone attached) and skin on.

This is an easy traybake and it is a meal in itself, or it can be bulked out with any of the extras (which can easily be prepped while the traybake cooks). The flavours only improve, so leftovers are great the next day (just keep them in an airtight container in the refrigerator overnight, then reheat gently in the oven until piping hot before serving).

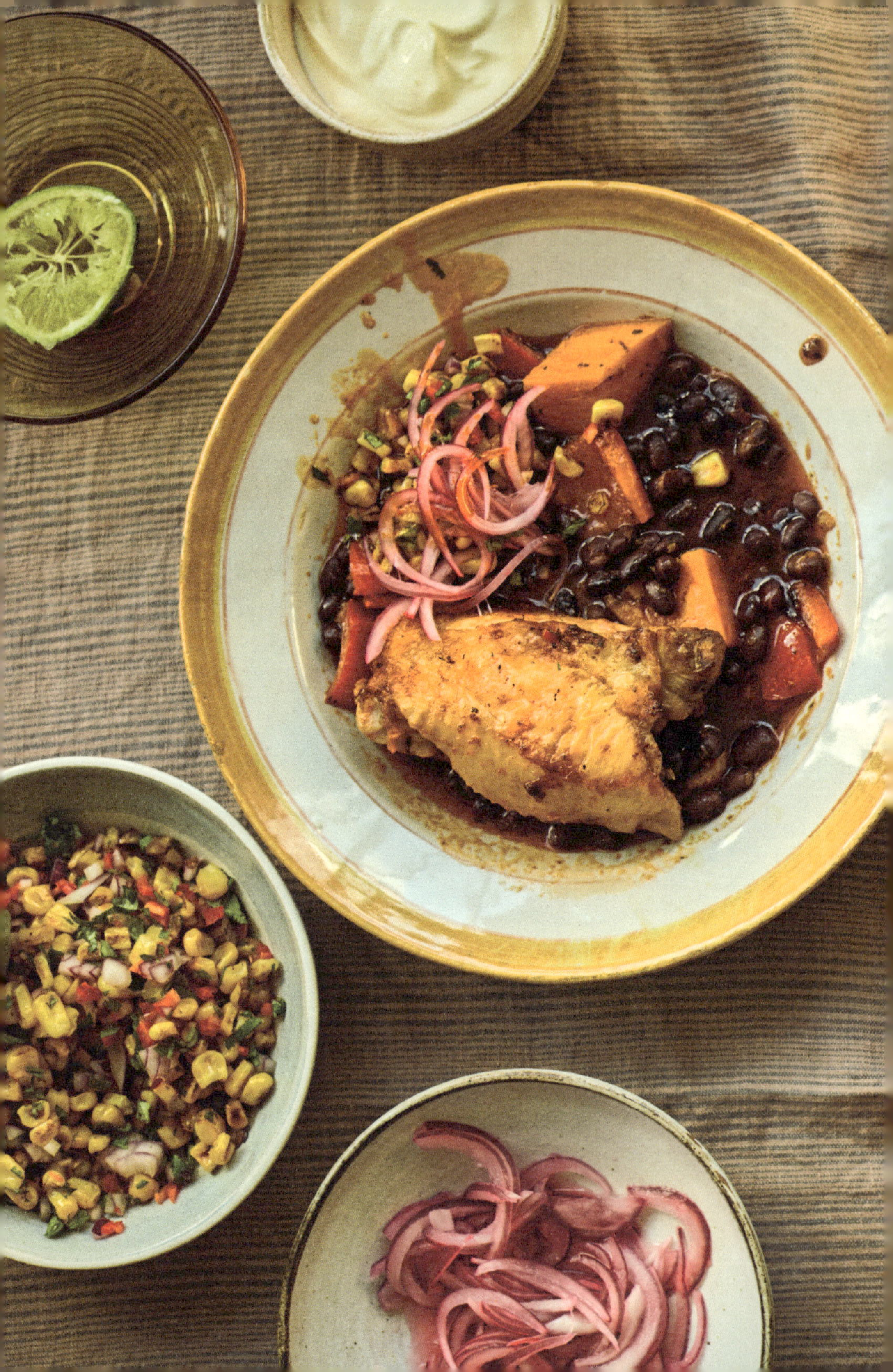

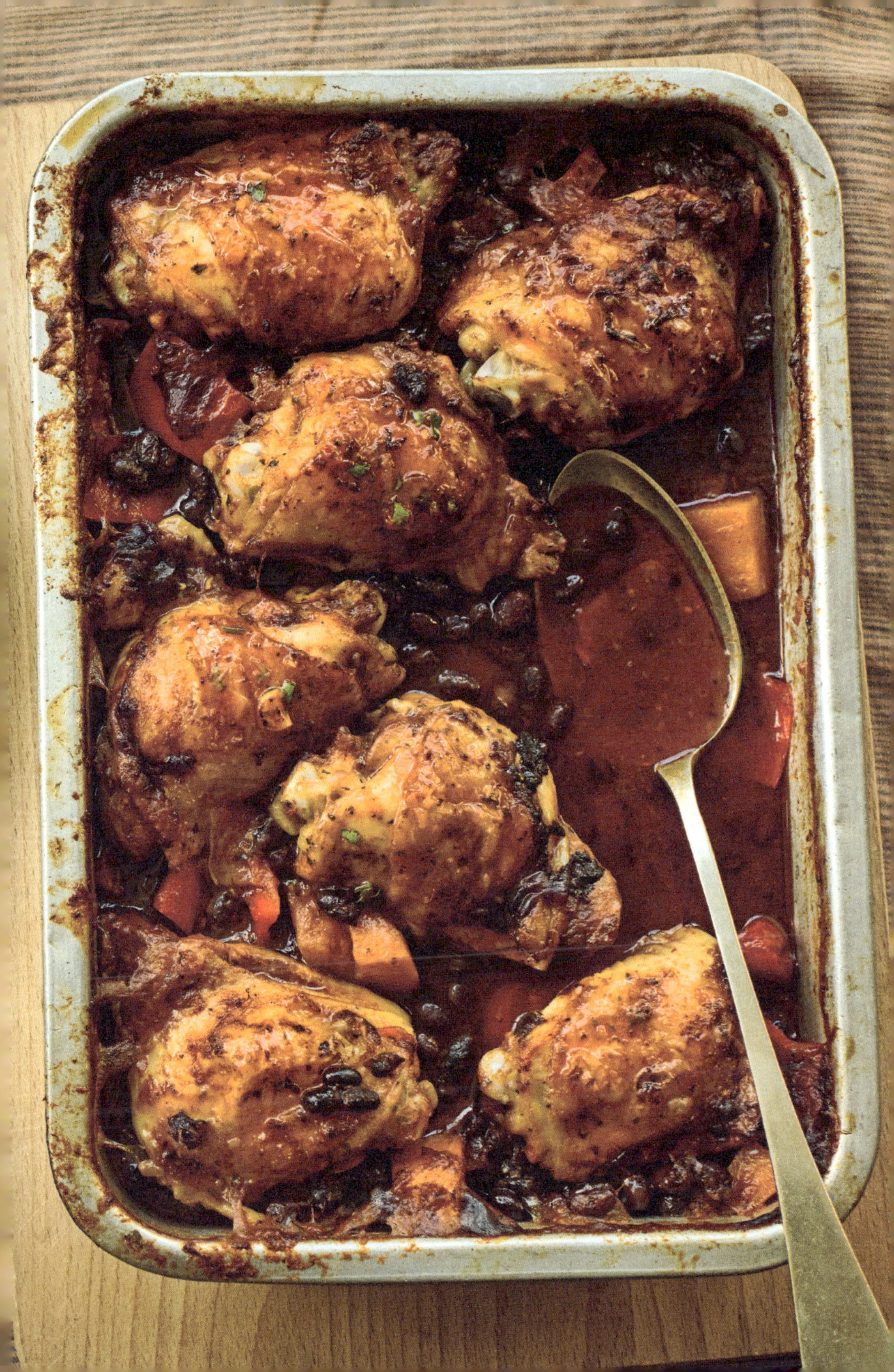

LONGEVITY 25 LARDER

SERVES 6

A dish with a huge Longevity Larder score! It achieves this with a combination of plenty of antioxidant-rich spices and anti-inflammatory ginger and turmeric, alongside cauliflower for vitamin K, and calcium-rich spinach, green beans and chickpeas.

cauliflower biryani

- 300g/10½oz white basmati rice
- 2 green cardamom pods, crushed
- 1 bay leaf
- 1 cinnamon stick
- 1 x 400g/14oz can chickpeas, drained and rinsed
- ½ cauliflower, cut into 4cm/1½in florets
- 1 pepper (red or green), deseeded and cut into 3cm/1¼in dice
- 150g/5½oz green beans, cut into 3cm/1¼in pieces
- 15g/½oz fresh ginger, peeled and finely grated
- 2 garlic cloves, crushed
- 1 green chilli, roughly chopped (deseeded if preferred)
- 2 tsp garam masala
- 1 tsp ground cumin
- ½ tsp ground cardamom
- 1 tsp ground coriander
- ½ tsp ground turmeric
- 1 tsp chilli powder (mild, medium or hot, as preferred)
- 150g/5½oz natural yogurt
- 2 tbsp lemon juice
- 300ml/10fl oz vegetable stock
- ½ tsp saffron strands, infused in 1 tbsp boiling water
- Salt and black pepper
- 30g/1oz flaked almonds or halved cashew nuts (or a mixture of both), lightly toasted (see Cook's Note on p.182), to finish

1. Cover the rice with cold water in a bowl and leave to soak for at least 30 minutes (see Cook's Notes, overleaf). Drain, rinse well (until the water runs clear) and then transfer to a saucepan, along with the cardamom pods, bay leaf and cinnamon stick. Cover with ample boiling water from the kettle, add ½ teaspoon of salt and simmer for about 7 minutes, until al dente. Drain well, mix with the chickpeas and set aside.

2. Preheat the oven to 220°C fan/475°F/Gas 9.

3. Spread the cauliflower, pepper and green beans out in a large, ovenproof sauté pan or casserole pan, about 30cm/12in wide, and set aside.

4. Place the ginger, garlic, chilli and ground spices in a food processor (or blender/Nutribullet) along with the yogurt, lemon juice, 2 teaspoons of salt and a good grind of black pepper. Blitz until smooth, then pour this over the vegetables and stir to combine.

recipe continues overleaf

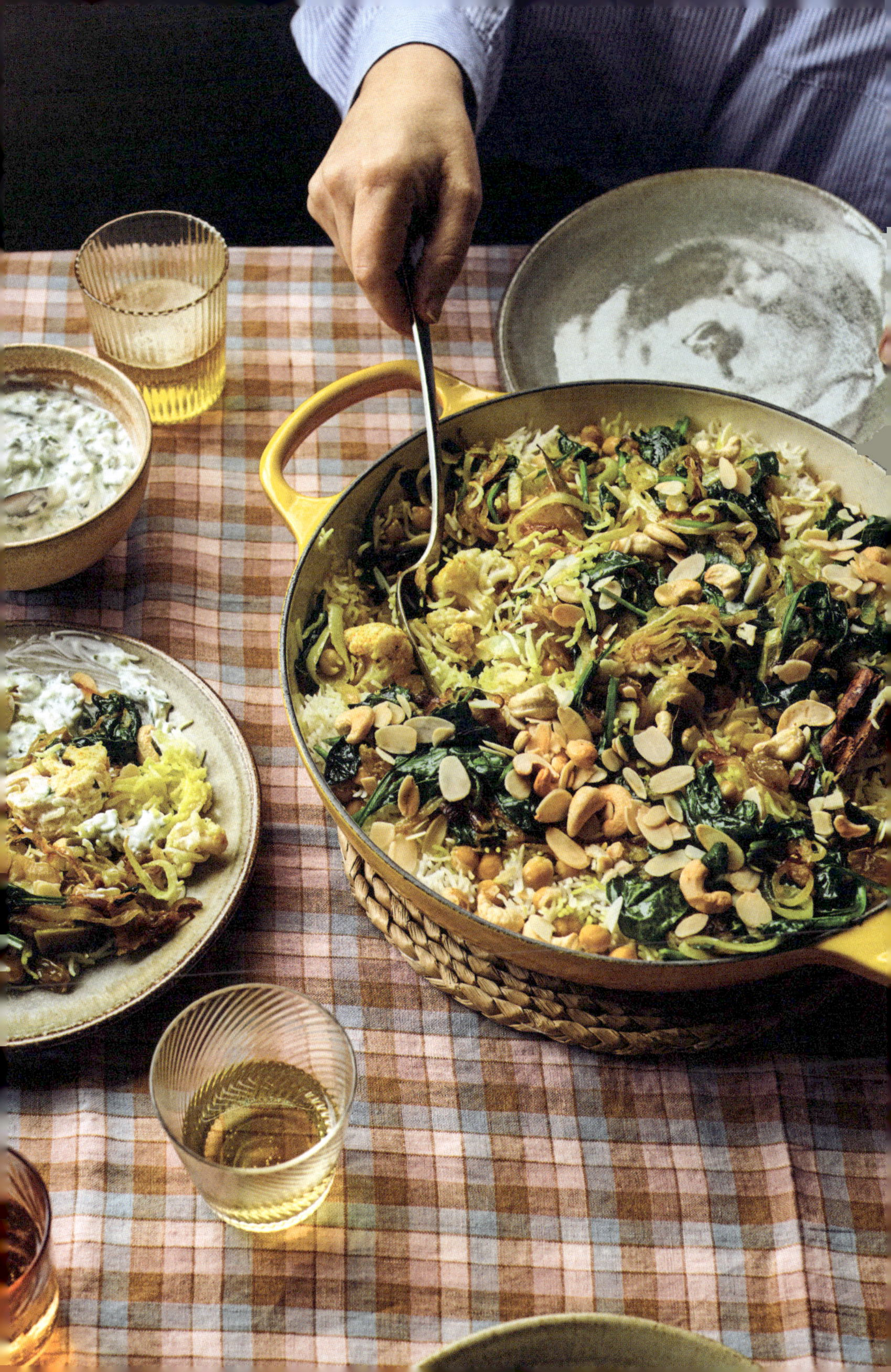

RAITA

150g/5½oz natural yogurt
½ cucumber, grated and squeezed-out
1 tbsp lemon juice
10g/¼oz fresh mint leaves, shredded
1 small garlic clove, crushed
½ tsp salt

CARAMELIZED ONIONS

3 tbsp olive (or coconut) oil
2 onions, thinly sliced
1 tsp ground cumin
½ tsp ground turmeric
120g/4¼oz baby spinach leaves
20g/¾oz golden sultanas (optional)

5. Roast for about 15 minutes, so that the vegetables soften and start to take on some colour. Remove the pan from the oven, reduce the oven temperature to 180°C fan/400°F/Gas 6 and spread the rice–chickpea mix out in an even layer on top of the vegetables; don't remove the whole aromatics – they are not to be eaten but they look lovely. Pour over the stock, followed by the saffron-infused water and seal the pan well – a layer of foil, as well as the lid, is the best way to ensure a tight seal. Bake for 30 minutes.

6. Meanwhile, in a small serving bowl, mix together all the ingredients for the raita. Cover and refrigerate until ready to use.

7. When the biryani is 20 minutes or so from being ready, cook the caramelized onions. Add the oil to a large frying or sauté pan and place over a medium-high heat. Add the onions and cook for about 15 minutes, until soft and golden, stirring often and reducing the heat to medium if they are catching. Add the cumin and turmeric, cook for a minute and then stir through the spinach and golden sultanas (if using). Cook for another couple of minutes, stirring to wilt the spinach.

8. Remove the biryani from the oven. Spoon the caramelized onion mixture evenly over the top of the biryani, sprinkle over the toasted nuts to finish and then serve with the raita spooned alongside.

COOK'S NOTES

Don't skip the soaking, draining and rinsing stage for the rice: fluffiness is what a good biryani is all about!

Don't be put off by the long list of ingredients for this recipe! It actually all comes together quite easily.

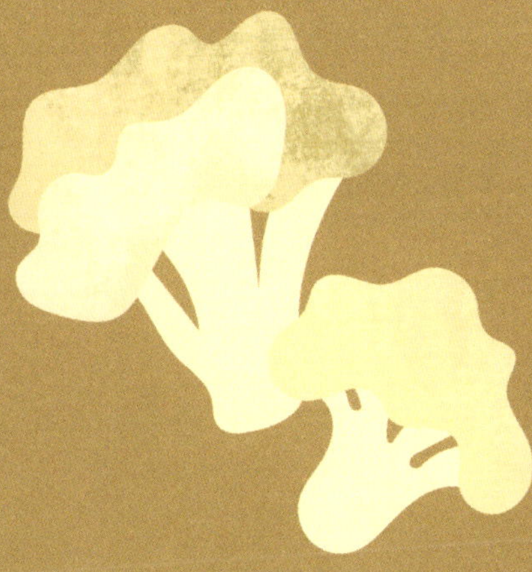

LONGEVITY 11 LARDER

SERVES 2

This is a far more nutritious alternative to shop-bought baked beans. Lycopene from the tomatoes helps to reduce oxidative stress and has been shown to have a potential protective effect against postmenopausal bone loss.[117] The Kale and Almond Pesto provides vitamin K, magnesium and calcium, alongside the polyphenols in the olive oil, and the cannellini beans provide a source of protein and minerals, too.

posh baked beans with feta and kale and almond pesto

400g/14oz cherry tomatoes
2 tbsp olive oil, plus extra for drizzling to serve
2 garlic cloves, left whole but slightly crushed with the side of a knife
A few sprigs of fresh oregano (optional)
1 x 570g/1lb 4½oz jar cannellini beans, drained and rinsed
2 slices of your favourite bread
2–3 tbsp Kale and Almond Pesto (see p.135)
Juice of ½ lemon
60g/2¼oz feta cheese
Salt and black pepper

1. Preheat the oven to 180°C fan/400°F/Gas 6.

2. Place the cherry tomatoes in an ovenproof dish, then add the olive oil, garlic and oregano (if using) and season with a pinch of salt and a good grind of black pepper. Give it a stir and then roast in the oven for 10 minutes.

3. Remove from the oven, add the cannellini beans, giving it all a good stir, then return to the oven for a final 5 minutes of cooking. The tomatoes should be blistering and collapsing. Discard the oregano stalks before serving.

4. Toast your bread.

5. Gently swirl the pesto and lemon juice through your baked beans, then pile onto your toast. Crumble the feta on top, drizzle with extra olive oil, then serve.

LONGEVITY 14 LARDER

SERVES 6

An ode to one of my favourite countries I have ever lived in, people- and food-wise – Vietnam. The markets were always brimming with different green leafy veg, and savoury food was eaten for every meal, including breakfast, unlike the ultra-processed foods we often eat.

This rice dish traditionally uses poached chicken, and the liquid is then used to cook the rice, with bowls of the liquor served on the side. But serving it platter-style makes it super family-friendly and creates less washing up, too. This is a very bright salad, reminiscent of the *bánh mì* you buy on the street there, made with anti-inflammatory supportive turmeric, beta carotene-rich carrots and capsaicin in the chilli. The herbs are also rich in antioxidants, magnesium, calcium and vitamins C and K.

hoi an-style chicken and carrot rice

CARROT SALAD

- 2 carrots, peeled and shaved with a vegetable peeler into long, thin strips
- 80ml/3fl oz rice wine vinegar
- ½ tsp salt
- 1 red chilli, deseeded and finely chopped
- 3 spring onions, white parts only, thinly sliced
- 10g/¼oz fresh coriander leaves, roughly chopped
- 10g/¼oz fresh mint leaves, roughly chopped
- 15g/½oz fresh Thai basil leaves, shredded

CHICKEN

- 2 tsp ground turmeric
- 20g/¾oz fresh ginger, peeled and finely grated
- 3 tbsp olive oil
- 1 large chicken (about 1.6kg/3lb 8oz)
- Salt and black pepper

1. Preheat the oven to 220°C fan/475°F/Gas 9.

2. For the carrot salad, put the carrots, vinegar and salt in a small bowl, massage together and leave to pickle for at least an hour.

3. For the chicken, in a small bowl, mix together the turmeric, ginger, olive oil, 1½ teaspoons of salt and a good grind of black pepper to make a paste. Rub this all over the chicken – on top of and under the skin. Place the chicken in a roasting tin and roast for 10 minutes. Reduce the oven temperature to 190°C fan/410°F/Gas 6½ and roast for another hour, basting a few times, until fully cooked through.

4. Meanwhile, make the marinade (see overleaf). Add the lime juice, sesame oil, fish sauce and olive oil to a large, heatproof bowl and set aside.

recipe continues overleaf

MARINADE
4 tbsp lime juice
2 tbsp sesame oil
2 tbsp Thai fish sauce
1 tbsp olive oil

TURMERIC RICE
300g/10½oz white basmati and wild rice mix
½ tsp ground turmeric
1 tsp salt
About 600ml/1 pint boiling water (or chicken stock)

CRISPY SHALLOTS
2 tbsp olive oil
2 shallots, thinly sliced

5. Remove the chicken from the oven and carefully pour the cooking juices (you should have about 120ml/4fl oz) into the bowl with the marinade. Set the chicken aside and, once cool enough to handle, tear the meat off the bones (see Cook's Notes) into large bite-sized chunks. Add the meat (and skin) to the bowl with the marinade, stir to mix and set aside while you cook the rice.

6. Add the rice, turmeric and salt to a saucepan and place over a medium heat. Dry-fry for a minute and then pour over the boiling water. Cook for about 25 minutes (or according to the packet instructions) until the rice is cooked through and all the water has been absorbed.

7. Meanwhile, heat the olive oil for the shallots in a small frying pan over a high heat. Add the sliced shallots and cook for 8–10 minutes, stirring a few times, until soft but crispy at the edges. Transfer onto a kitchen paper-lined plate and set aside.

8. Drain the pickled carrots, then add them to a bowl with the remaining salad ingredients and toss together gently to mix.

9. Spread the rice out on a large platter and arrange the marinated chicken on top. Spoon over any remaining marinade and then spoon the carrot salad over the top. Finish with the fried shallots.

COOK'S NOTES

Shop-bought crispy fried shallots are a useful thing to have in the pantry and save the work of frying the shallots here.

Thinly sliced radishes (around 80g/3oz) make a nice addition.

You can use the chicken carcass to make stock for another recipe.

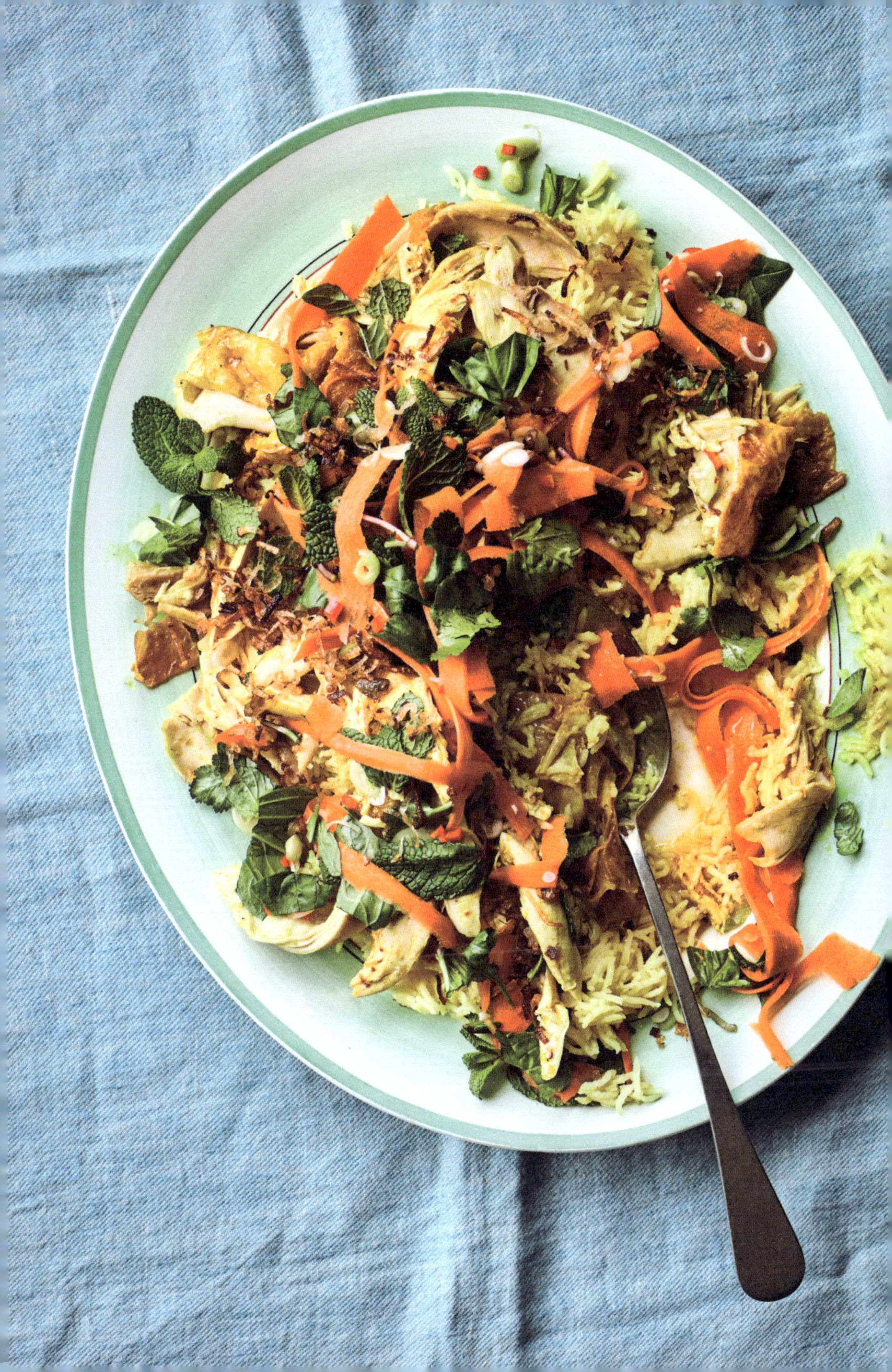

LONGEVITY 14 LARDER

SERVES 4

A dish combining phytoestrogen-rich tofu, two ways, alongside dill and parsley, which provide bone-supporting nutrients such as magnesium, manganese, phosphorus and calcium, alongside antioxidants vitamin C and K.

sesame-crusted tofu and herb-packed greens

TOFU–TAHINI SAUCE

150g/5½oz silken tofu, drained
2 tbsp tahini
1 tsp tamari
1 tsp maple syrup (or runny honey)

HERB-PACKED GREENS

4 tbsp olive oil
1 onion, thinly sliced
2 garlic cloves, crushed
2 tsp ground cumin
1 tsp ground cinnamon
50g/1¾oz fresh dill, roughly chopped
50g/1¾oz fresh parsley, roughly chopped
150–200ml/5–7fl oz hot vegetable stock (or water)
500g/1lb 2oz mixed greens (such as kale, cavolo nero and chard), hard stems removed and leaves roughly chopped (400g/14oz prepped weight)
Salt and black pepper

1. Add all the ingredients for the tofu–tahini sauce to a blender, blitz until smooth, then set aside.

2. For the greens, add the olive oil to a large sauté pan and place over a medium heat. Add the onion and cook for about 8 minutes, stirring a few times, until the edges are starting to crisp up. Add the garlic, ground spices, ½ teaspoon of salt and some black pepper and cook for a couple of minutes before adding the herbs.

3. Cook for 5 minutes, stirring often, adding in a splash of the stock if things are starting to catch. Add the greens, in batches, and cook for a final 10 minutes, adding more stock, as needed, until the greens are all soft and there is no liquid left in the pan.

recipe continues overleaf

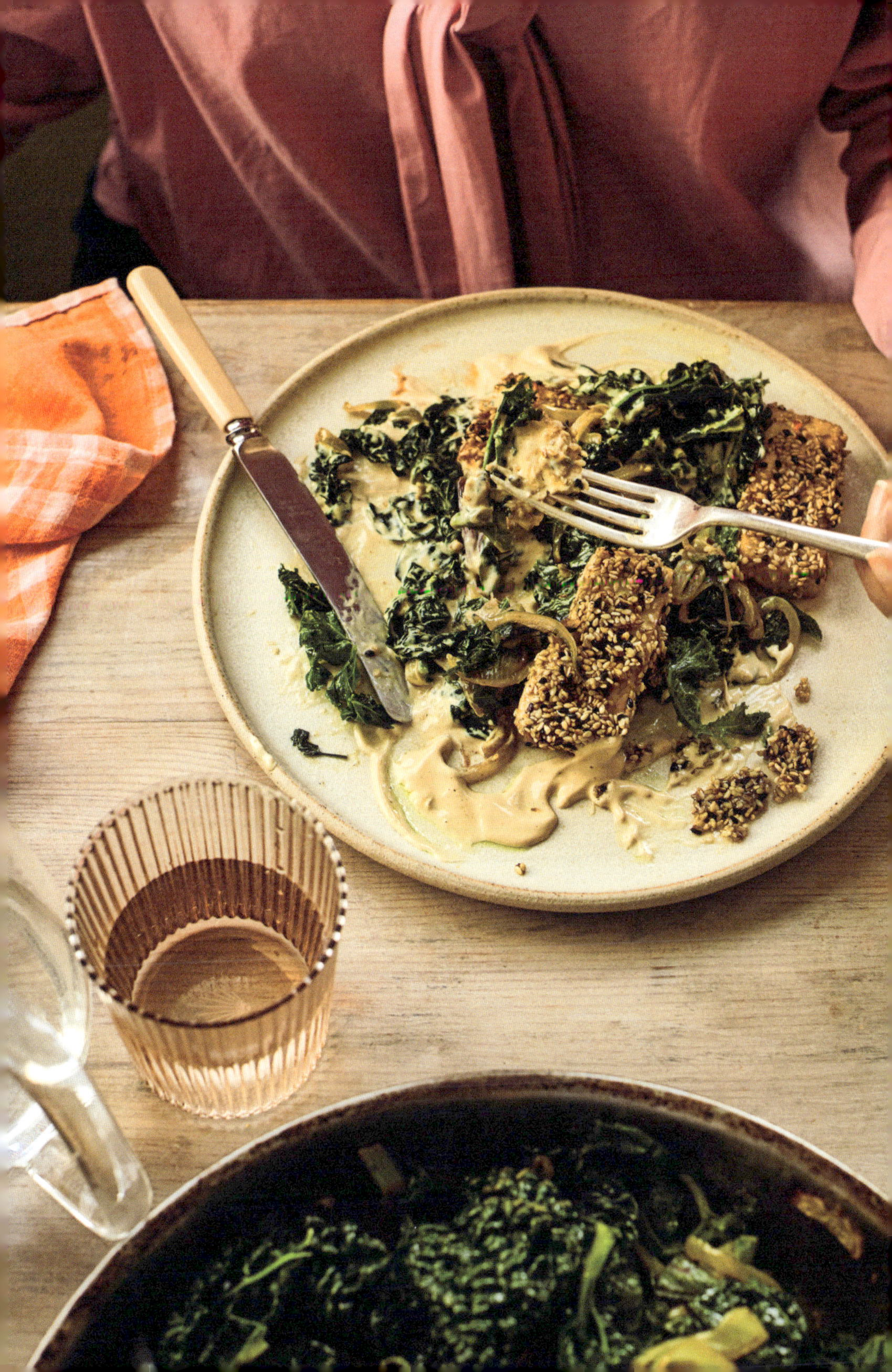

FRIED TOFU

2 x 300g/10½oz blocks of extra-firm tofu, cut into 1cm/½in-thick rectangles
2 tbsp cornflour
2 tbsp tamari
100g/3½oz sesame seeds (a mix of white and black looks great)
About 4 tbsp rapeseed (or other neutral) oil, for frying

4. Meanwhile, toss the tofu in the cornflour to coat, followed by the tamari and then the sesame seeds, pressing them so that they stick to the tofu. Heat the oil in a frying pan over a medium-high heat. Add the tofu and cook for about 4 minutes, turning so that all sides get cooked – once ready, it will look lovely and golden-crusted.

5. To serve, spread the tofu–tahini sauce out on a large serving plate or platter and spoon the warm greens on top. Top with the fried tofu and serve.

COOK'S NOTES

Taking time to cook the herbs and greens down is a great way of ramping up the flavour. Fresh coriander also works well in place of one of the herbs listed – just keep the weight the same.

Both the tofu–tahini sauce and the herb-packed greens can be made ahead of time, but the fried tofu is best straight out of the pan. The sauce will keep in an airtight container in the refrigerator for up to 3 days. The greens can be cooked as above, then cooled and refrigerated in an airtight container for up to 2 days. Reheat gently in a pan until piping hot before serving (they will lose a bit of their vibrant green colour, but will still taste great).

uk–us cooking terms:

- Aubergine – eggplant
- Beetroot – beet
- Bicarbonate of soda – baking soda
- Borlotti bean – cranberry bean
- Broad bean – fava bean
- Butter bean – lima bean
- Cannellini bean – white bean/white kidney bean
- Celeriac – celery root
- Chickpea – garbanzo bean
- Chicory – endive
- Chilli flakes – crushed red pepper/red pepper flakes
- Coriander (leaves) – cilantro
- Cornflour – cornstarch
- Courgette – zucchini
- French beans – string/green beans
- Grill – boil/broiler
- Globe artichoke – French artichoke
- Pepper – bell pepper/capsicum
- Prawn – shrimp
- Puy lentils – French green lentils
- Rapeseed (oil) – canola
- Rocket – arugula
- Spring onions – green onions/scallions
- Sweetcorn – corn/maize
- Tomato purée – tomato paste

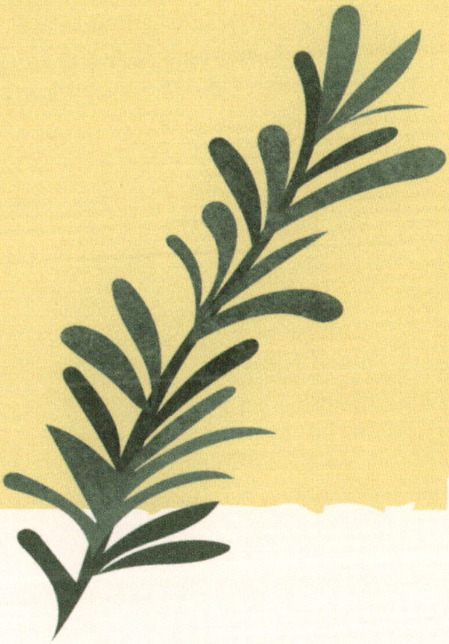

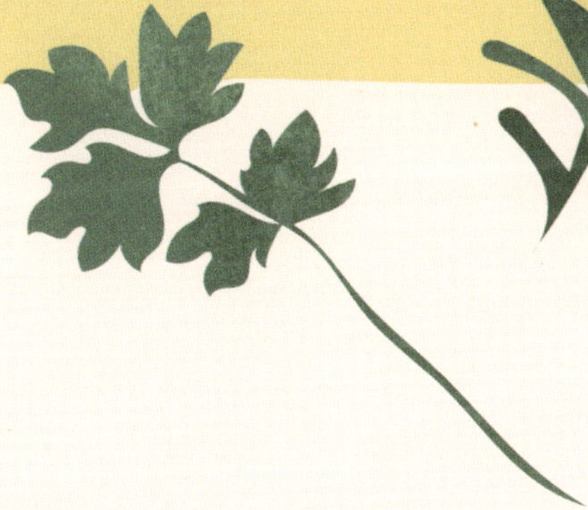

references

POST-MENOPAUSE AS THE GATEWAY TO OPTIMAL AGEING

1 https://www.ons.gov.uk/peoplepopulationandcommunity/birthsdeathsandmarriages/lifeexpectancies/bulletins/nationallifetablesunitedkingdom/2021to2023additionaldata

2 https://www.gov.uk/government/publications/mortality-insights-from-gad-december-2024

3 Fadnes, L.T., Økland, J.-M., Haaland, Ø.A., and Johansson K.A. 'Estimating impact of food choices on life expectancy: A modeling study', *PLoS Medicine* (2022), 19(2): e1003889. https://doi.org/10.1371/journal.pmed.1003889

4 Aliberti, S.M., Capunzo, M., and Funk, R.H.W. 'Systems and molecular biology of longevity and preventive medicine: Brain-energy–microbiome–exposome synergies in Blue Zones and the Cilento case', *International Journal of Molecular Science* (2025), 26: 7887. https://doi.org/10.3390/ijms26167887

5 López-Otín, C., Blasco, M.A., Partridge, L., Serrano, M., and Kroemer, G. 'Hallmarks of aging: An expanding universe', *Cell* (2023), 186(2): 243–278, ISSN 0092-8674. https://doi.org/10.1016/j.cell.2022.11.001

6 McCarthy, M., and Raval, A.P. 'The peri-menopause in a woman's life: A systemic inflammatory phase that enables later neurodegenerative disease', *Journal of Neuroinflammation* (2020), 17(317). https://doi.org/10.1186/s12974-020-01998-9

7 Zhao, Y., and Liu, Y.-S. 'Longevity factor FOXO3: A key regulator in aging-related vascular diseases', *Frontiers in Cardiovascular Medicine* (2021), 8:778674. doi: 10.3389/fcvm.2021.778674

8 Pereira, Q.C., Dos Santos, T.W., Fortunato, I.M., and Ribeiro, M.L. 'The molecular mechanism of polyphenols in the regulation of ageing hallmarks', *International Journal of Molecular Science* (14 Mar 2023), 24(6): 5508. doi: 10.3390/ijms24065508. PMID: 36982583; PMCID: PMC10049696.

9 Parrotta, M.E., Colangeli, L., Scipione, V., Vitale, C., Sbraccia, P., and Guglielmi, V. 'Time restricted eating: A valuable alternative to calorie restriction for addressing obesity?', *Current Obesity Reports* (3 Feb 2025), 14(1): 17. doi: 10.1007/s13679-025-00609-z. PMID: 39899119; PMCID: PMC11790783.

10 Baechle, J.J., Chen, N., Makhijani, P., Winer, S., Furman, D., and Winer, D.A. 'Chronic inflammation and the hallmarks of aging', *Molecular Metabolism* (Aug 2023), 74: 101755. doi: 10.1016/j.molmet.2023.101755. Epub 15 June 2023. PMID: 37329949; PMCID: PMC10359950.

11 Ames, B.N., Atamna, H., and Killilea, D.W. 'Mineral and vitamin deficiencies can accelerate the mitochondrial decay of aging', *Molecular Aspects of Medicine* (Aug–Oct 2055), 26(4–5): 363–78. doi: 10.1016/j.mam.2005.07.007. PMID: 16102804.

12 Shannon, O.M., *et al.* 'Mediterranean diet and the hallmarks of ageing', *European Journal of Clinical Nutrition* (2021), 75: 1176–92. https://doi.org/10.1038/s41430-020-00841-x

13 Davinelli, S., Trichopoulou, A., Corbi, G., De Vivo, I., and Scapagnini, G. 'The potential nutrigeroprotective role of Mediterranean diet and its functional components on telomere length dynamics', *Ageing Research Reviews* (2019), 49: 1–10, ISSN 1568-1637. https://doi.org/10.1016/j.arr.2018.11.001

14 Estruch, R., *et al.* 'Primary prevention of cardiovascular disease with a Mediterranean diet supplemented with extra-virgin olive oil or nuts', *New England Journal of Medicine* (2018), 378: e34. https://www.nejm.org/doi/full/10.1056/NEJMoa1800389

15 Salas-Salvadó, J., *et al.* 'Reduction in the incidence of type 2 diabetes with the Mediterranean diet: Results of the PREDIMED-Reus nutrition intervention randomized trial', *Diabetes Care* (2011), 34: 14–19. https://pubmed.ncbi.nlm.nih.gov/20929998/

16 Klimova, B., Novotny, M, Schlegel, P., and Valis, M. 'The effect of Mediterranean diet on cognitive functions in the elderly population', *Nutrients* (16 June 2021), 13(6): 2067. doi: 10.3390/nu13062067. PMID: 34208741; PMCID: PMC8235742.

17 Calcabrini, C., *et al.* 'Protective effect of *Juglans regia* L. walnut extract against oxidative DNA damage', *Plant Foods for Human Nutrition* (2017), 72: 192–97. https://doi.org/10.1007/s11130-017-0609-2

18 Silva-Soto, M.Á., *et al.* 'Extra virgin olive oil phenolic compounds: Modulating mitochondrial function and protecting against chronic diseases – a narrative review', *Nutrients* (25 Apr 2025), 17(9): 1443. doi: 10.3390/nu17091443. PMID: 40362752; PMCID: PMC12073407.

19 Willcox, B.J., Willcox, D.C., Todoriki, H., Fujiyoshi, A., Yano, K., He, Q., Curb, J.D., and Suzuki, M. 'Caloric restriction, the traditional Okinawan diet, and healthy aging: The diet of the world's longest-lived people and its potential impact on morbidity and life span', *Annals of the New York Academy of Sciences* (Oct 2007), 1114: 434–55. doi: 10.1196/annals.1396.037. PMID: 17986602.

20 Nestor, M.S., Bhupalam, V., Awad, N., and Hetzel, J.D. 'The therapeutic role of genistein in perimenopausal and postmenopausal women', *Journal of Clinical and Aesthetic Dermatology* (Oct 2024), 17(10):45–53. PMID: 39445324; PMCID: PMC11495164.

21 Min, B.R., Marsh, L.E., Brathwaite, K., and Daramola, A.O. 'Effects of tissue culture and mycorrhiza applications in organic farming on concentrations of phytochemicals and antioxidant capacities in ginger (*Zingiber officinale* Roscoe) rhizomes and leaves', *Journal of Food Science* (Apr 2017), 82(4): 873–81. doi: 10.1111/1750-3841.13661. Epub 23 Feb 2017. PMID: 28231393.

22 Cerri, L., Parri, S., Dias, M.C., Fabiano, A., Romi, M., Cai, G., Cantini, C., and Zambito, Y. 'Olive leaf extracts from three Italian olive cultivars exposed to drought stress differentially protect cells against oxidative stress', *Antioxidants* (Basel; 7 Jan 2024), 13(1): 77. doi: 10.3390/antiox13010077. PMID: 38247501; PMCID: PMC10812426.

23 Pereira, Q.C., Dos Santos, T.W., Fortunato, I.M., and Ribeiro, M.L. 'The molecular mechanism of polyphenols in the regulation of ageing hallmarks', *International Journal of Molecular Science* (14 Mar 2023), 24(6):5508. doi: 10.3390/ijms24065508. PMID: 36982583; PMCID: PMC10049696.

24 Sarubbo, F., Moranta, D., Tejada, S., Jiménez, M., and Esteban, S. 'Impact of gut microbiota in brain ageing: Polyphenols as beneficial modulators', *Antioxidants* (2023), 12: 812. https://doi.org/10.3390/antiox12040812

25 D'Angelo, S. 'Diet and aging: The role of polyphenol-rich diets in slow down the shortening of telomeres: A review', *Antioxidants* (Basel; 7 Dec 2023), 12(12): 2086. doi: 10.3390/antiox12122086. PMID: 38136206; PMCID: PMC10740764.

26 Chuang, S.C., *et al.* 'Fiber intake and total and cause-specific mortality in the European prospective investigation into cancer and nutrition cohort', *American Journal of Clinical Nutrition* (July 2012), 96(1): 164–74. doi: 10.3945/ajcn.111.028415. Epub 30 May 2012. PMID: 22648726.

27 Reynolds, A., Mann, J., Cummings, J., Winter, N., Mete, E., and Te Morenga, L. 'Carbohydrate quality and human health: A series of systematic reviews and meta-analyses', *Lancet* (2 Feb 2019), 393(10170): 434–45. doi: 10.1016/S0140-6736(18)31809-9. Epub 10 Jan 2019. Erratum in: *Lancet*, 2 Feb 2019, 393(10170): 406. doi: 10.1016/

28 Ragonnaud, E., and Biragyn, A. 'Gut microbiota as the key controllers of "healthy" aging of elderly people', *Immun Ageing* (2021), 18: 2. https://doi.org/10.1186/s12979-020-00213-w

29 Makki, K., Deehan, E.C., Walter, J., and Bäckhed, F. 'The impact of dietary fiber on gut microbiota in host health and disease', *Cell Host & Microbe* (2018), 23(6): 705–15. https://pubmed.ncbi.nlm.nih.gov/29902436/

30 Zheng, L., Jia, Z., Gong, S., Zheng, T., Zhuang, Y., Lin, L., Li, Q., Lin, F., and Ren, M. 'Dietary rhythms and biological aging risk across multiple organs', *npj Science of Food* (2026). https://doi.org/10.1038/s41538-026-00799-3

METABOLIC HARMONY

31 Mosconi, L., *et al.* 'Menopause impacts human brain structure, connectivity, energy metabolism, and amyloid-beta deposition', *Scientific Reports* (2021), 11: 10867. https://doi.org/10.1038/s41598-021-90084-y

32 Hadi, A., Askarpour, M., Salamat, S., Ghaedi, E., Symonds, M.E., Miraghajani, M. 'Effect of flaxseed supplementation on lipid profile: An updated systematic review and dose-response meta-analysis of sixty-two randomized controlled trials', *Pharmacological Research*, (2020), 152: 04622, ISSN 1043-6618. https://doi.org/10.1016/j.phrs.2019.104622

33 https://www.bhf.org.uk/what-we-do/news-from-the-bhf/news-archive/2016/august/women-are-50-per-cent-more-likely-than-men-to-be-given-incorrect-diagnosis-following-a-heart-attack

34 Rippe, J.M. 'Lifestyle strategies for risk factor reduction, prevention, and treatment of cardiovascular disease', *American Journal of Lifestyle Medicine* (2 Dec 2018), 13(2): 204–12. doi: 10.1177/1559827618812395. PMID: 30800027; PMCID: PMC6378495.

35 McCarthy, M., and Raval, A.P. 'The peri-menopause in a woman's life: A systemic inflammatory phase that enables later neurodegenerative disease' *Journal of Neuroinflammation* (23 Oct 2020), 17(1): 317. doi: 10.1186/s12974-020-01998-9. PMID: 33097048; PMCID: PMC7585188.

36 Sorriento, D., and Iaccarino, G. 'Inflammation and cardiovascular diseases: The most recent findings', *International Journal of Molecular Science* (9 Aug 2019), 20(16): 3879. doi: 10.3390/ijms20163879. PMID: 31395800; PMCID: PMC6719998.

37 Tasić, T., Tadić, M., and Lozić, M. 'Hypertension in women', *Frontiers in Cardiovascular Medicine* (3 June 2022), 9: 905504. doi: 10.3389/fcvm.2022.905504. PMID: 35722103; PMCID: PMC9203893.

38 De Oliveira-Gomes, D., Joshi, P.H., Peterson, E.D., Rohatgi, A., Khera, A., and Navar A.M. 'Apolipoprotein B: Bridging the gap between evidence and clinical practice', *Circulation* (2 July 2024), 150(1): 62–79. doi: 10.1161/CIRCULATIONAHA.124.068885. Epub 1 July 2024. PMID: 38950110; PMCID: PMC11219008.

39 https://www.bhf.org.uk/research-projects/investigationof-the-mechanisms-underlying-the-vasodilator-effects-of-the-n3-pufas-fish-oils

40 Guasch-Ferré, M., Liu, X., Malik, V.S., Sun, Q., Willett, W.C., Manson, J.E., Rexrode, K.M., Li, Y., Hu, F.B., and Bhupathiraju, S.N. 'Nut consumption and risk of cardiovascular disease', *Journal of the American College of Cardiology* (14 Nov 2017), 70(20): 2519–32. doi: 10.1016/j.jacc.2017.09.035. PMID: 29145952; PMCID: PMC5762129.

41 Ros, E., Martínez-González, M.A., Estruch, R., Salas-Salvadó, J., Fitó, M., Martínez, J.A., and Corella, D. 'Mediterranean diet and cardiovascular health: Teachings of the PREDIMED study', *Advances in Nutrition* (14 May 2014), 5(3): 330S-6S. doi: 10.3945/an.113.005389. PMID: 24829485; PMCID: PMC4013190.

42 Ferrari, C.K.B. 'Anti-atherosclerotic and cardiovascular protective benefits of Brazilian nuts', *Frontiers in Bioscience* (scholar edition; 1 Jan 2020), 12(1): 38–56. doi: 10.2741/S539. PMID: 31585864.

43 https://www.sciencedirect.com/topics/agricultural-and-biological-sciences/platelet-aggregation

44 Cox, F.F., Misiou, A., Vierkant, A., Ale-Agha, N., Grandoch, M., Haendeler, J., and Altschmied, J. 'Protective effects of curcumin in cardiovascular diseases—Impact on Oxidative Stress and Mitochondria', *Cells* (20 Jan 2022), 11(3): 342. doi: 10.3390/cells11030342. PMID: 35159155; PMCID: PMC8833931.

45 Ockermann, P., Headley, L., Lizio, R., and Hansmann, J. 'A review of the properties of anthocyanins and their influence on factors affecting cardiometabolic and cognitive health', *Nutrients* (18 Aug 2021), 13(8): 2831. doi: 10.3390/nu13082831. PMID: 34444991; PMCID: PMC8399873.

46 Stull, A.J., *et al.* 'The state of the science on the health benefits of blueberries: A perspective', *Frontiers in Nutrition* (11 June 2024), 11: 1415737. doi: 10.3389/fnut.2024.1415737. PMID: 38919390; PMCID: PMC11196611.

47 Almeida, C., Gonçalves-Nobre, J.G., Aplium Costa, D., and Barata, P. 'The potenital links between human gut microbiota and cardiovascular health and disease – Is there a gut–cardiovascular axis?' *Frontiers in Gastroenterology* (2023), 2: 1235126. doi: 10.3389/fgstr.2023.1235126

48 Murphy, K., O'Donovan, A.N., Caplice, N.M., Ross, R.P., and Stanton, C. 'Exploring the gut microbiota and cardiovascular disease', *Metabolites* (29 July 2021), 11(8): 493. doi: 10.3390/metabo11080493. PMID: 34436434; PMCID: PMC8401482.

49 Cheng, H.M., Koutsidis, G., Lodge, J.K., Ashor, A.W., Siervo, M., and Lara, J. 'Lycopene and tomato and risk of cardiovascular diseases: A systematic review and meta-analysis of epidemiological evidence', *Critical Reviews in Food Science and Nutrition* (2019), 59(1): 141–58.

doi: 10.1080/10408398.2017.1362630. Epub 25 Sep 2017. PMID: 28799780.

50 Imaizumi, V.M., Laurindo, L.F., Manzan, B., Guiguer, E.L., Oshiiwa, M., Otoboni, A.M.M.B., Araujo, A.C., Tofano, R.J., and Barbalho, S.M. 'Garlic: A systematic review of the effects on cardiovascular diseases', *Critical Reviews in Food Science and Nutrition* (2023), 63(24): 6797–819. doi: 10.1080/10408398.2022.2043821. Epub 23 Feb 2022. PMID: 35193446.

51 Gulati, A., Banker, H., Muhammad, A.A., Anamika, F., and Jain, R. 'Unlocking the potential: Phytoestrogens and cardiovascular health', *Current Cardiology Reviews* (2025), 21(3): e1573403X333952. doi: 10.2174/011573403X333952241203050033. PMID: 39757642; PMCID: PMC12172217.

52 Sekikawa, A., Ihara, M., Lopez, O., Kakuta, C., Lopresti, B., Higashiyama, A., Aizenstein, H., Chang, Y.F., Mathis, C., Miyamoto, Y., Kuller, L., and Cui, C. 'Effect of S-equol and soy isoflavones on heart and brain', *Current Cardiology Reviews* (2019), 15(2): 114–35. doi: 10.2174/1573403X15666181205104717. PMID: 30516108; PMCID: PMC6520578.

53 DiNicolantonio, J.J., Liu, J., and O'Keefe, J.H. 'Magnesium for the prevention and treatment of cardiovascular disease', *Open Heart* (1 Jul 2018), 5(2): e000775. doi: 10.1136/openhrt-2018-000775. PMID: 30018772; PMCID: PMC6045762.

54 Morelli, M.B., Gambardella, J., Castellanos, V., Trimarco, V., and Santulli, G. 'Vitamin C and cardiovascular disease: An update', *Antioxidants* (Basel; 3 Dec 2020), 9(12): 1227. doi: 10.3390/antiox9121227. PMID: 33287462; PMCID: PMC7761826.

55 Bendinelli, B., *et al.* 'Fruit, vegetables, and olive oil and risk of coronary heart disease in Italian women: The EPICOR study', *American Journal of Clinical Nutrition* (2011), 9(2), 2011: 275–83, ISSN 0002-9165. https://doi.org/10.3945/ajcn.110.000521

56 Naghedi, A., Haghaninejad, H., Varastehravan, H., Naghedi, A., and Farshadi, N. 'Effect of vitamin D supplements on left ventricular ejection fraction in patients with heart failure: A systematic review and meta-analysis of randomized controlled trials', *Revista Portuguesa de Cardiologia* (English edition; 2021), 40(6): 447–55, ISSN 2174-2049. https://doi.org/10.1016/j.repce.2021.07.010

57 Bazzano, L.A., Thompson, A.M., Tees, M.T., Nguyen, C.H., and Winham, D.M. 'Non-soy legume consumption lowers cholesterol levels: A meta-analysis of randomized controlled trials', *Nutrition, Metabolism and Cardiovascular Diseases* (Feb 2011), 21(2): 94–103. doi: 10.1016/j.numecd.2009.08.012. Epub 25 Nov 2009. PMID: 19939654; PMCID: PMC2888631.

58 Thorisdottir, B., Arnesen, E.K., Bärebring, L., Dierkes, J., Lamberg-Allardt, C., Ramel, A., Nwaru, B.I., Söderlund, F., and Åkesson, A. 'Legume consumption in adults and risk of cardiovascular disease and type 2 diabetes: A systematic review and meta-analysis', *Food and Nutrition Research* (30 May 2023), 67. doi: 10.29219/fnr.v67.9541. PMID: 37288088; PMCID: PMC10243120.

59 Reiners, S., Hebestreit, S., Wedekind, L., Kiehntopf, M., Klink, A., Rummler, S., Glei, M., Lorkowski, S., Schlörmann, W., and Dawczynski, C. 'Effect of a regular consumption of traditional and roasted oat and barley flakes on blood lipids and glucose metabolism–A randomized crossover trial', *Frontiers in Nutrition* (2 Feb 2023), 10: 1095245. doi: 10.3389/fnut.2023.1095245. PMID: 36819683; PMCID: PMC9932717.

60 Laukkanen, T., Khan, H., Zaccardi, F., and Laukkanen, J.A. 'Association between sauna bathing and fatal cardiovascular and all-cause mortality events', *JAMA Internal Medicine* (Apr 2015), 175(4): 542–8. doi: 10.1001/jamainternmed.2014.8187. PMID: 25705824

BRAIN FOOD

61 Maki, P.M., and Weber, M.T. 'A research primer for studies of cognitive changes across the menopause transition', *Climacteric* (Aug 2021), 24(4): 382–88. doi: 10.1080/13697137.2021.1905625. PMID: 34240671.

62 Dhana, K., Evans, D.A., Rajan, K.B., Bennett, D.A., and Morris, M.C. 'Healthy lifestyle and the risk of Alzheimer dementia: Findings from 2 longitudinal studies', *Neurology* (28 July 2020), 95(4): e374–e383. doi: 10.1212/WNL.0000000000009816. Epub 17 June 2020. PMID: 32554763; PMCID: PMC7455318.

63 Baker, L.D., *et al.* 'Structured vs self-guided multidomain lifestyle interventions for global cognitive function: The US POINTER randomized clinical trial', *JAMA* (2025), 334(8): 681–91. doi:10.1001/jama.2025.12923

64 Marengoni, A., Rizzuto, D., Fratiglioni, L., Antikainen, R., Laatikainen, T., Lehtisalo, J., Peltonen, M., Soininen, H., Strandberg, T., Tuomilehto, J., Kivipelto, M., and Ngandu, T. 'The effect of a 2-year intervention consisting of diet, physical exercise, cognitive training, and monitoring of vascular risk on chronic morbidity—The FINGER randomized controlled trial', *Journal of the American Medical Directors Association* (Apr 2018), 19(4): 355–60.e1. doi: 10.1016/j.jamda.2017.09.020. Epub 3 Nov 2017. PMID: 29108888

65 Lehtisalo, J., Rusanen, M., Solomon, A., Antikainen, R., Laatikainen, T., Peltonen, M., Strandberg, T., Tuomilehto, J., Soininen, H., Kivipelto, M., and Ngandu, T. 'Effect of a multi-domain lifestyle intervention on cardiovascular risk in older people: the FINGER trial', *European Heart Journal* (1 June 2022), 43(21): 2054–61. doi: 10.1093/eurheartj/ehab922. PMID: 35051281; PMCID: PMC9156384.

66 Sekikawa, A., Ihara, M., Lopez, O., Kakuta, C., Lopresti, B., Higashiyama, A., Aizenstein, H., Chang, Y.F., Mathis, C., Miyamoto, Y., Kuller, L., and Cui, C. 'Effect of S-equol and soy isoflavones on heart and brain', *Current Cardiology Reviews* (2019), 15(2): 114–35. doi: 10.2174/1573403X15666181205104717. PMID: 30516108; PMCID: PMC6520578.

67 Sekikawa, A., Wharton, W., Butts, B., Veliky, C.V., Garfein, J., Li, J., Goon, S., Fort, A., Li, M., and Hughes, T.M. 'Potential protective mechanisms of S-equol, a metabolite of soy isoflavone by the gut microbiome, on cognitive decline and dementia', *International Journal of Molecular Science* (7 Oct 2022), 23(19): 11921. doi: 10.3390/ijms231911921. PMID: 36233223; PMCID: PMC9570153.

68 Wang, Y., Hernandez, G., Mack, W.J., Schneider, L.S., Yin, F., and Brinton, R.D. 'Retrospective analysis of phytoSERM for management of menopause-associated vasomotor symptoms and cognitive decline: A pilot study on pharmacogenomic effects of mitochondrial haplogroup and APOE genotype on therapeutic efficacy', *Menopause* (Jan 2020), 27(1): 57–65. doi: 10.1097/GME.0000000000001418. PMID: 31567873; PMCID: PMC7100617.

69 Wang, Y., Shang, Y., Mishra, A., Bacon, E., Yin, F., and Brinton, R. 'Midlife chronological and endocrinological transitions in brain metabolism: System biology basis for increased Alzheimer's risk in female brain', *Scientific Reports* (22 May 2020), 10(1): 8528. doi: 10.1038/s41598-020-65402-5. PMID: 32444841; PMCID: PMC7244485.

70 Wang. J.-H., Guo, L., Wang, S., Yu, N.-W., and Guo, F.-Q. 'The potential pharmacological mechanisms of β-hydroxybutyrate for improving cognitive functions', *Current Opinion in Pharmacology* (2022), 62: 15–22, ISSN 14714892. www.sciencedirect.com/science/article/pii/S1471489221001582

71 Maki, P.M., and Thurston, R.C. 'Menopause and brain health: Hormonal changes are only part of the story', *Frontiers in Neurology* (23 Sep 2020), 11: 562275. doi: 10.3389/fneur.2020.562275. PMID: 33071945; PMCID: PMC7538803.

72 Capasso, L., De Masi, L., Sirignano, C., Maresca, V., Basile, A., Nebbioso, A., Rigano, D., and Bontempo, P. 'Epigallocatechin gallate (EGCG): Pharmacological properties, biological activities and therapeutic potential', *Molecules* (1 Feb 2025), 30(3): 654. doi: 10.3390/molecules30030654. PMID: 39942757; PMCID: PMC11821029.

73 Zhang, M., and Tang, Z. 'Therapeutic potential of natural molecules against Alzheimer's disease via SIRT1 modulation', *Biomedicine & Pharmacotherapy* (2023) 161: 114474, ISSN 0753-3322. https://doi.org/10.1016/j.biopha.2023.114474

74 *ibid*

75 Tzekaki, E.E., Tsolaki, M., Geromichalos, G.D., and Pantazaki, A.A. 'Extra virgin olive oil consumption from mild cognitive impairment patients attenuates oxidative and nitrative stress reflecting on the reduction of the PARP levels and DNA damage', *Experimental Gerontology* (2021), 156: 111621, ISSN 0531-5565. https://doi.org/10.1016/j.exger.2021.111621

76 O'Brien, J., Okereke, O., Devore, E., Rosner, B., Breteler, M., and Grodstein, F. 'Long-term intake of nuts in relation to cognitive function in older women', *Journal of Nutrition, Health and Aging* (May 2014), 18(5): 496–502. doi: 10.1007/s12603-014-0014-6. PMID: 24886736; PMCID: PMC4105147.

77 Ros, E., Martínez-González, M.A., Estruch, R., Salas-Salvadó, J., Fitó, M., Martínez, J.A., and Corella, D. 'Mediterranean diet and cardiovascular health: Teachings of the PREDIMED study', *Advances in Nutrition* (14 May 2014), 5(3): 330S-6S. doi: 10.3945/an.113.005389. PMID: 24829485; PMCID: PMC4013190.

78 Terock, J., Bonk, S., Frenzel, S., Wittfeld, K., Garvert, L., Hosten, N., Nauck, M., Völzke, H., Van der Auwera, S., and Grabe, H.J. 'Vitamin D deficit is associated with accelerated brain aging in the general population', *Psychiatry Research: Neuroimaging* (2022), 327: 111558, ISSN 0925-4927, https://doi.org/10.1016/j.pscychresns.2022.111558

79 Mazza E., Fava A., Ferro Y., Moraca M., Rotundo S., Colica C., Provenzano F., Terracciano R., Greco M., Foti D., Gulletta E., Russo D., Bosco D., Pujia A., and Montalcini T. 'Impact of legumes and plant proteins consumption on cognitive performances in the elderly', *Journal of Translational Medicine* (22 May 2017), 15(1): 109. doi: 10.1186/s12967-017-1209-5. PMID: 28532453; PMCID: PMC5440936.

80 Yeh, T.S., Yuan, C., Ascherio, A., Rosner, B.A., Blacker, D., and Willett, W.C. 'Long-term dietary protein intake and subjective cognitive decline in US men and women', *American Journal of Clinical Nutrition* (11 Jan 2022), 115(1): 199–210. doi: 10.1093/ajcn/nqab236. PMID: 34293099; PMCID: PMC8755047.

81 Li, Y., Li, Y., Gu, X., Liu, Y., Dong, D., Kang, J.H., Wang, M., Eliassen, H., Willett, W.C., Stampfer, M.J., and Wang, D. 'Long-term intake of red meat in relation to dementia risk and cognitive function in US adults', *Neurology* (11 Feb 2025), issue 104 (3): e210286. https://doi.org/10.1212/WNL.000000000021028

82 Reddy, P.H., *et al.* 'Protective effects of Indian spice curcumin against amyloidβ in Alzheimer's disease', *Journal of Alzheimer's Disesase* (2018), 61(3): 843–66. doi: 10.3233/JAD-170512. PMID: 29332042; PMCID: PMC5796761.

83 Miranda, M., Morici, J.F., Zanoni, M.B., and Bekinschtein, P. 'Brain-derived neurotrophic factor: A key molecule for memory in the healthy and the pathological brain', *Frontiers in Cellular Neuroscience* (7 Aug 2019), 13: 363. doi: 10.3389/fncel.2019.00363. PMID: 31440144; PMCID: PMC6692714.

84 Liu, H., Deng, Y., Chen, L., Weng, S., and Xu, D. 'The effect of omega 3 supplementation on serum brain-derived neurotrophic factor: A systematic review and meta-analysis', *European Journal of Integrative Medicine* (2023), 61: 102264, ISSN 1876-3820. https://doi.org/10.1016/j.eujim.2023.102264

85 Terock, J., Bonk, S., Frenzel, S., Wittfeld, K., Garvert, L., Hosten, N., Nauck, M., Völzke, H., Van der Auwera, S., and Grabe, H.J. 'Vitamin D deficit is associated with accelerated brain aging in the general population', *Psychiatry Research: Neuroimaging* (2022), 327: 111558, ISSN 0925-4927. https://doi.org/10.1016/j.pscychresns.2022.111558

86 Seidler, K., and Barrow, M. 'Intermittent fasting and cognitive performance – Targeting BDNF as potential strategy to optimise brain health', *Frontiers in Neuroendocrinology* (2022), 65: 100971, ISSN 0091-3022. https://doi.org/10.1016/j.yfrne.2021.100971

87 Kalt, W., Cassidy, A., Howard, L.R., Krikorian, R., Stull, A.J., Tremblay, F., and Zamora-Ros, R. 'Recent research on the health benefits of blueberries and their anthocyanins', *Advances in Nutrition* (1 Mar 2020), 11(2): 224–36. doi: 10.1093/advances/nmz065. PMID: 31329250; PMCID: PMC7442370.

88 Clarke, K.M., Etemadmoghadam, S., Danner, B., Corbett, C., Ghaseminejad-Bandpey, A., Dopler, M., Parker-Garza, J., Alhneif, M., Babu, S., Ogunbona, O.B., Gonzalez, A.D., Salardini, A., and Flanagan, M.E. 'The Nun Study: Insights from 30 years of aging and dementia research', *Alzheimer's and Dementia* (Feb 2025), 21(2): e14626. doi: 10.1002/alz.14626. PMID: 39998266; PMCID: PMC11852352.

89 Aktan Süzgün, M., Tang, Q., and Stefani, A. 'Sleep abnormalities and risk of Alzheimer's disease', *Current Neurology and Neuroscience Reports* (13 Oct 2025), 25(1): 67. doi: 10.1007/s11910-025-01451-5. PMID: 41082137; PMCID: PMC12518432.

UNBREAKABLE

90 Nestor, M.S., Bhupalam, V., Awad, N., and Hetzel, J.D. 'The therapeutic role of genistein in perimenopausal and postmenopausal women', *Journal of Clinical and Aesthetic Dermatology* (Oct 2024), 17(10): 45–53. PMID: 39445324; PMCID: PMC11495164.

91 Atteritano, M., Mazzaferro, S., Frisina, A., Cannata, M.L., Bitto, A., D'Anna, R., Squadrito, F., Macrì, I., Frisina, N., and Buemi, M. 'Genistein effects on quantitative ultrasound parameters and bone mineral density in osteopenic postmenopausal women', *Osteoporosis International* (Nov 2009), 20(11): 1947–54. doi: 10.1007/s00198-009-0883-4. Epub 24 Feb 2009. PMID: 19238303.

92 Mangano, K.M., Sahni, S., and Kerstetter, J.E. 'Dietary protein is beneficial to bone health under conditions of adequate calcium intake:

An update on clinical research', *Current Opinion in Clinical Nutrition and Metabolic Care* (Jan 2014), 17(1): 69–74. doi: 10.1097/MCO.0000000000000013. PMID: 24316688; PMCID: PMC4180248.

93 Sun, C., Yang, A., Teng, F., and Xia, Y. 'Efficacy of collagen peptide supplementation on bone and muscle health: A meta-analysis', *Frontiers in Nutrition* (18 Sep 2025), 12: 1646090. doi: 10.3389/fnut.2025.1646090. PMID: 41049371; PMCID: PMC12488437.

94 Genuis, S.J., and Bouchard, T.P. 'Combination of Micronutrients for Bone (COMB) Study: Bone density after micronutrient intervention', *Journal of Environmental and Public Health* (2012), 354151. doi:10.1155/2012/354151

95 Feskanich, D., Weber, P., Willett, W.C., Rockett, H., Booth, S.L., and Colditz, G.A. 'Vitamin K intake and hip fractures in women: A prospective study', *American Journal of Clinical Nutrition* (Jan 1999), 69(1): 74–79. doi: 10.1093/ajcn/69.1.74. PMID: 9925126.

96 Haghighat, M.M.L., Haghpanah, B., and Milajerdi, A. 'Dietary vitamin K intake and fracture risk: A systematic review and dose-response meta-analysis on the interplay with Vitamin D', *Current Rheumatology Reviews* (9 Sep 2025). doi: 10.2174/0115733971393704250828112958.PMID: 40947710.

97 Guo, J., Zhou, Z., Gong, J., Hu, W., and Liu, Y. 'Vitamin K intake levels are associated with bone health in people aged over 50 years: A NHANES-based survey', *Frontiers in Medicine* (2024), 11:1485095. doi: 10.3389/fmed.2024.1485095

98 Khazai, N., Judd, S.E., and Tangpricha, V. 'Calcium and vitamin D: Skeletal and extraskeletal health', *Current Rheumatology Reports* (Apr 2008), 10(2): 110–17. doi: 10.1007/s11926-008-0020-y. PMID: 18460265; PMCID: PMC2669834.

99 Morris, M.C., Wang, Y., Barnes, L.L., Bennett, D.A., Dawson-Hughes, B., and Booth, S.L. 'Nutrients and bioactives in green leafy vegetables and cognitive decline: Prospective study', *Neurology* (16 Jan 2018), 90(3): e214–e222. doi: 10.1212/WNL.0000000000004815. Epub 20 Dec 2017. PMID: 29263222; PMCID: PMC5772164.

100 Melguizo-Rodríguez, L., Manzano-Moreno, F.J., Illescas-Montes, R., Ramos-Torrecillas, J., Luna-Bertos, E., Ruiz, C., and García-Martínez, O. 'Bone protective effect of extra-virgin olive oil phenolic compounds by modulating osteoblast gene expression', *Nutrients* (25 July 2019), 11(8): 1722. doi: 10.3390/nu11081722. PMID: 31349732; PMCID: PMC6722737.

101 Andreo-López, M.C., Contreras-Bolívar, V., García-Fontana, B., García-Fontana, C., and Muñoz-Torres, M. 'The influence of the Mediterranean dietary pattern on osteoporosis and sarcopenia', *Nutrients* (20 July 2023), 15(14): 3224. doi: 10.3390/nu15143224. PMID: 37513646; PMCID: PMC10385532.

102 Bai, B., Xie, X., Yue, Y., Cui, J., Xie, F., and Yao, F. 'Association between immune-inflammatory index and osteoporosis: A systematic review and meta-analysis', *European Journal of Medical Research* (16 July 2025), 30(1): 632. doi: 10.1186/s40001-025-02893-w. PMID: 40665418; PMCID: PMC12265382.

103 Liu, Z., Cai, S., Chen, Y., Peng, Z., Jian, H., Zhang, Z., and Huang, H. 'The association between dietary omega-3 intake and osteoporosis: A NHANES cross-sectional study', *Frontiers in Nutrition* (10 Jan 2025), 11: 1467559. doi: 10.3389/fnut.2024.1467559. PMID: 39867554; PMCID: PMC11757016.

104 Docherty, S., Doughty, F.L., and Smith, E.F. 'The acute and chronic effects of lion's mane mushroom supplementation on cognitive function, stress and mood in young adults: A double-blind, parallel groups, pilot study', *Nutrients* (20 Nov 2023), 15(22): 4842. doi: 10.3390/nu15224842. PMID: 38004235; PMCID: PMC10675414.

105 Chen, Y., Wang, X., Zhang, C., Liu, Z., Li, C., and Ren, Z. 'Gut microbiota and bone diseases: A growing partnership'. *Frontiers in Microbiology* (6 May 2022), 13: 877776. doi: 10.3389/fmicb.2022.877776. PMID: 35602023; PMCID: PMC9121014

106 Zdzieblik, D., Oesser, S., and König, D. 'Specific bioactive collagen peptides in osteopenia and osteoporosis: Long-term observation in postmenopausal women', *Journal of Bone Metabolism* (Aug 2021), 28(3): 207–13. doi: 10.11005/jbm.2021.28.3.207. Epub 31 Aug 2021. PMID: 34520654; PMCID: PMC8441532.

DEVELOPING LONG-TERM LONGEVITY RITUALS

107 Bowler, D.E., *et al.* 'A systematic review of evidence for the added benefits to health of exposure to natural environments', *BMC Public Health* (2010), 10: 456. https://doi.org/10.1186/1471-2458-10-456

108 Magrone, T., Russo, M.A., and Jirillo, E. 'Cocoa and dark chocolate polyphenols: From biology to clinical applications', *Frontiers in Immunology* (2017) 8:677. doi: 10.3389/fimmu.2017.00677

109 Daniele, A., Lucas, S.J.E., and Rendeiro, C. 'Dietary flavanols preserve upper- and lower-limb endothelial function during sitting in high- and low-fit young healthy males', *Journal of Physiology* (2025), https://doi.org/10.1113/JP289038

110 Bajaj, A., John-Henderson, N.A., Cundiff, J.M., Marsland, A.L., Manuck, S.B., and Kamarck, T.W. 'Daily social interactions, close relationships, and systemic inflammation in two samples: Healthy middle-aged and older adults', *Brain, Behavior, and Immunity* (Nov 2016), 58: 152–64. doi: 10.1016/j.bbi.2016.06.004. Epub 8 June 2016. PMID: 27288715; PMCID: PMC7526085.

111 Lehmiller, J.J., Graham, C.A., Ferrall, L., Mendelson, E.A., and Prine, M.S. 'The role of masturbation in relieving symptoms associated with menopause', *Menopause* (1 Apr 2026), 33(4):384–94; doi: 10.1097/GME.0000000000002675

112 Jeffery, G., Fosbury, R., Barrett, E., Hogg, C., Carmona, M.R., and Powner, M.B. 'Longer wavelengths in sunlight pass through the human body and have a systemic impact which improves vision'. *Scientific Reports* (8 July 2025), 15(1): 24435. doi: 10.1038/s41598-025-09785-3. PMID: 40628952; PMCID: PMC12238558.

THE RECIPES

113 Domènech, M., Serra-Mir, M., Roth, I., Freitas-Simoes, T., Valls-Pedret, C., Cofán, M., López, A., Sala-Vila, A., Calvo, C., Rajaram, S., Sabaté, J., and Ros, E. 'Effect of a walnut diet on office and 24-hour ambulatory blood pressure in elderly individuals', *Hypertension* (May 2019), 73(5): 1049–57. doi: 10.1161/HYPERTENSIONAHA.118.12766. PMID: 30879358; PMCID: PMC6467552.

114 Torres-Oteros, D., *et al.* 'Unveiling the impact of peanut consumption on telomere length in young and healthy individuals: Insights from the ARISTOTLE Study: A randomized clinical trial', *Antioxidants* (2025), 14: 467. https://doi.org/10.3390/antiox14040467

115 Delaney, K., Tsang, M., Kern, M., Rayo, V.U., Jason, N., Hong, M.Y., Liu, C., and Hooshmand, S. 'Strawberries modestly improve cognition and cardiovascular health in older adults', *Nutrition, Metabolism, and Cardiovascular Diseases* (Aug 2025), 35(8): 104018. doi: 10.1016/j.numecd.2025.104018. Epub 18 Mar 2025. PMID: 40199714.

116 Lyu, C., Jacques, P.F., Doraiswamy, P.M., Young, B., Gurnani, A.S., Au, R., and Hwang, P.H. 'Flavonoid-rich fruit intake in midlife and late-life and associations with risk of dementia: The Framingham Heart Study. *Journal of Prevention of Alzheimer's Disease* (2024), 11(5): 1270–79. doi: 10.14283/jpad.2024.116. PMID: 39350372; PMCID: PMC11436402.

117 Walallawita, U.S., Wolber, F.M., Ziv-Gal, A., Kruger, M.C., and Heyes, J.A. 'Potential role of lycopene in the prevention of postmenopausal bone loss: Evidence from molecular to clinical studies', *International Journal of Molecular Science* (27 Sep 2020), 21(19): 7119. doi: 10.3390/ijms21197119. PMID: 32992481; PMCID: PMC7582596.

index

acknowledgements

To my husband Jules and my two sons, Oscar and Sam. You are always such an amazing support. Boys, you know a lot about menopause and beyond now, too, so I hope this will mean that you will empathize with and cook for your girlfriends, wives and friends when they reach this stage, like your Dad does for me.

Thank you to my editor Lucy Smith and designer Lily Wilson for being such a pleasure to work with again.

Thank you to the hugely talented illustrator Maggie Stephenson, who completely got the brief and who created the serene women who now grace the front cover, as well as the beautiful food for the Longevity Larder – I think these would make a great wallpaper!

Tara Wigley, you make magic with my recipes and I thank you, friend, for your skills, your focus on testing every detail, your appetite (eating the best part of the entire Hoi An-style chicken!) and for being such an utter delight to work with again.

Thank you to my sage contributors Kate Codrington, Joyce Harper, Melinda McDougall, Suzy Reading and Dinah Siman. Thank you for all the work you do to support and inspire us as we navigate midlife and beyond. And to the brilliant Rachel de Thample, whose work on fermentation and medicinal tonics I have admired for many years.

The photoshoot brought together the special circle of women that I was lucky enough to work with on my first cookbook: Laura Edwards behind the lens, food stylist Rosie Ramsden, prop stylist Tabitha Hawkins, cookery and food prep by Georgia Rudd, and assistant photographers Phoebe Pearson and Jo Cowan. The shoot days went by in a flash as we busily talked while working – about growing children, love, art, travel, TV, grief (one of my oldest friends had recently died, so there were tears) and laughter – as well as feasting on the food that is within the pages of this book. I heard breaking news of the spring awakening of Tabitha's mother's pet tortoise Henry, who she's had for over 70 years. And now, Tabitha tells me, everything is right with the world. And even though we know it isn't, in that moment it felt like it could be. A joyful microcosm of womanhood, squeezed into two days.

about the author

Karen Newby is a nutritionist, speaker, food activist, author and regular media contributor. She holds a BSc in Nutritional Medicine and has over 15 years of clinical experience. She works extensively with women navigating menopause and post-menopause, translating complex nutritional science into practical, sustainable strategies that support long-term vitality. She is the author of two other books on the menopause: *The Natural Menopause Method* and *The Natural Menopause Method Cookbook*. Through her writing, Karen combines clinical expertise with practical recipes and lifestyle guidance, with an emphasis on preventative health. Having lived for many years in China and Vietnam, she has witnessed first-hand how traditional food cultures place nourishment front and centre of everyday life in contrast to the ultra-processed food culture prevalent in the UK, where she now lives. Karen is on a mission to help women reclaim agency over their health at menopause – through what they eat, how they live, by drawing on the wisdom of traditional food practices passed down by women from different cultures around the world. She champions a life free from a fear of ageing, so that post-menopausal lives can be vibrant, purposeful and fulfilling.

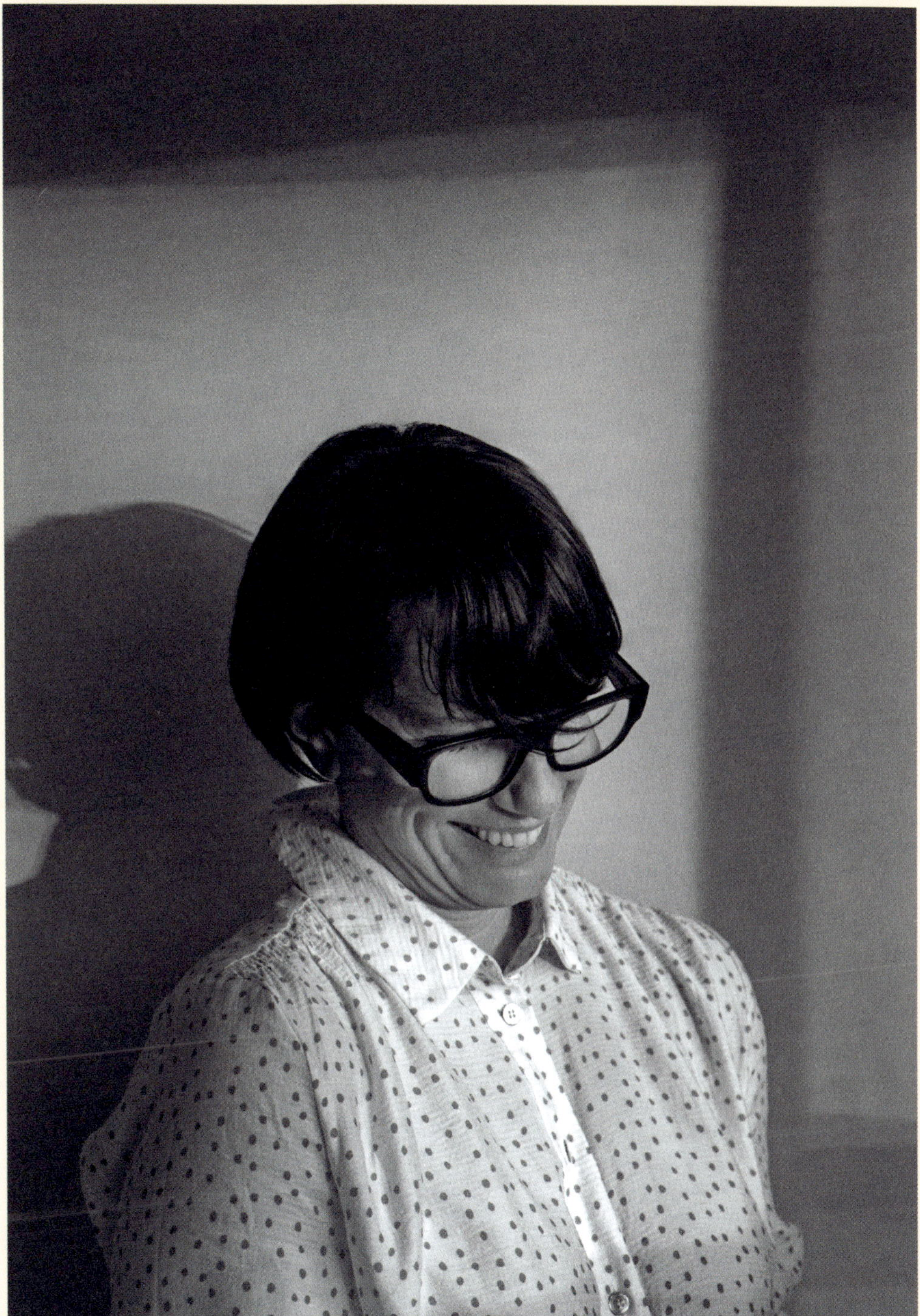

For Jules, Oscar and Sam – thank you for all the love.

Pavilion
An imprint of HarperCollins*Publishers* Ltd
1 London Bridge Street
London SE1 9GF

www.harpercollins.co.uk

HarperCollins*Publishers*
Macken House
39/40 Mayor Street Upper,
Dublin 1
D01 C9W8
Ireland

10 9 8 7 6 5 4 3 2 1

First published in Great Britain by Pavilion
An imprint of HarperCollins*Publishers* 2026

Karen Newby asserts the moral right
to be identified as the author of this work.
A catalogue record of this book is available
from the British Library.

ISBN 9780008818708

Publishing Director: Laura Russell
Commissioning Editor: Lucy Smith
Editorial Assistants: Daisy Gudmunsen
and Abigail Muth
Designer: Lily Wilson
Production Controller: Grace O'Byrne
Photographer: Laura Edwards
Photography Assistant: Phoebe Pearson
Food Stylist: Rosie Ramsden
Food Stylist Assistant: Georgia Rudd
Prop Stylist: Tabitha Hawkins
Artworker: James Boast
Illustrator: Maggie Stephenson
Proofreader: Angela Koo
Indexer: Lisa Footitt
Reproduction: Rival Colour Ltd, UK

Printed and bound by Papercraft in Malaysia

WHEN USING KITCHEN APPLIANCES
PLEASE ALWAYS FOLLOW THE
MANUFACTURER'S INSTRUCTIONS

MIX
Paper | Supporting
responsible forestry
FSC
www.fsc.org
FSC® C007207